"They say laughter is the best medicine, but I have never been sure of how to prescribe it until now. Read this book! Kat's anecdotes will make you smile as she attempts to stay positive and centered in our tumultuous, stressed out world."

— Dr. M., Physician

"The Happy Hypochondriac is hilarious, refreshing and uplifting. Spitzer tells a relatable, engaging story while making readers feel better about their own worries. Buy this book for the worrier in your life, or if you just want a good laugh."

— Dr. Marcus Jones, Professor, U.S. Naval Academy

"I, for one am thrilled that this book has been published. Mainly because now I can point to something actually in print to say 'SEE! This is what I live with!' But beyond its immense personal value to me in garnering the sympathy of family, friends, and random strangers on the street, this book is a realistic, funny, and heartwarming account of my wife's struggles with her, um, affliction. Readers will see reflections of themselves or loved-ones in these stories and find them inspiring and instructive. And maybe, just maybe, through this book, some other spouses of hypochondriacs may be able to get the sympathy they too so richly deserve."

— HHH (Happy Hypochondriac Husband)

D0723648

# The Happy Hypochondriac

# The Happy Hypochondriac

## Kat Spitzer

Baltimore, MD
www.apprenticehouse.com

Cover and internal design by: Eric Weinstein

Printed in the United States of America

ISBN: 978-1-934074-72-5
First Edition

Published by Apprentice House
The Future of Publishing...Today!

Apprentice House
Communication Department
Loyola University Maryland
4501 N. Charles Street
Baltimore, MD 21210

410.617.5265
410.617.2198 (fax)
www.ApprenticeHouse.com
info@ApprenticeHouse.com

*For my family.*

# Acknowledgments

I would like to thank my husband who told me I should write what I know and suggested I think about dealing with my "little problem." He was right (which is now permanently in print). I want to thank my kids who kept telling me I could do it, and show me all the time that they are as proud of me as I am of them. I would like to thank my mom, dad and sister for being such an interesting and inspiring family. I think of this book as a little love note to them. Many thanks to all the friends who have believed in me from the beginning and to all the readers who have supported me in my blog and other writings.

I extend a most heartfelt thanks to Kevin Atticks, Gregg Wilhelm and the students associated with Apprentice House who believed in the Happy Hypochondriac and thought others in the world might want to read it, too.

Thank you to all of the many doctors, nurses, therapists, medicines, strangers (and my friends and family again) for humoring me and aiding me through all of my worries and issues. You made me able to put the "Happy" before the hypochondriac. Jason, Jacob, Rachel, Kaitlyn, Britt, Laurie, Alan, Barbara, Sarah, Uncle Billy, Heavenly, my fabulous cousins, Jaime, Paul, Sasha, Melissa, James, Katie, Mary, Tracy, Jessica, Jenn and Brian, Pat, Dick and Barb, Christina, Kristin, Kristen, Sharon, Allyson, Karen, Michelle, Ann, Ryan, Dave, Amy, Cathy, Luna, Sadie; you all have given me so much love, help, and advice and shared in many of my little and big "traumas." Also, thank you to all those people in my life who inspired me in writing these stories. I love you all.

Hypochondriac Lesson #1:
If everyone's already laughing at you,
you might as well laugh at yourself.

## 1-When the World Gets Scary, Just Dance
### (Or, Early Indications I Might be a Hypochondriac)

I am blind. Where just moments ago I saw the sizzling flash of sequins like a bonfire at a Girl Scout camp out, I now see nothing. I am living my biggest nightmare where all the lights go out and nobody can hear me scream. Like the old woman, Mrs. Fletcher, in the medical alarm TV ad, I've fallen and I can't get up. She maybe broke a hip. I've broken my head. And I'm not old like her. I'm only a kid. I still have all my teeth. I think. Since I can't see, I don't know if blood or teeth or limbs are splattered all around me. Now that I consider the situation, I can't hear anything either. It sounds like I have my ear up to a large conch shell; just a loud and unnerving whooshing. It seems to ebb and flow with my heart beat. That can't be good. Is there anybody out there that can help me? Curse Eugenia for letting me fall. If she ever comes to my house for a sleepover, her underwear is going in the freezer first.

"And jazz hands. Jazz hands. Big. Wide. Jazz hands. I want to see a rainbow of sparkle coming off of those fingertips, girls." Clap, clap. "And stop." Kirk, our guest instructor with the skin of a hot dog beginning to glisten on a roller cooker, glanced over at our teacher and shrugged. We were a lost cause. Even his mid-level expertise -he thought he should've been a Broadway choreographer, but instead he taught children in suburban Orlando- could not crack this group. But his oversized pink sweatshirt with the silk-screened white cat on the front certainly made us smile the whole time. Who wears that besides grandmas? While the other classes of little girls always looked constipated with concentration, our group had the widest grins this side of a Miss America pageant. Our teachers should rejoice that we didn't laugh out loud while performing with that shirt in the room.

Miss Prudence looked over the class with a disapproving eye, one plucked eyebrow arched as she tapped her finger to her lip, gracefully sweeping her pointed foot around her body distractedly; just like a dancer should, according to the movies I'd seen. It was the eighties, and Miss Prudence personified Olivia Newton John's "Let's Get Physical" from head to toe. A terry cloth headband adorned the frosted tips of her hair, while a magenta leotard and thick, shiny, royal blue leggings, hugged her petite frame. The leotard had the high-cut leg that we all thought made us look slimmer but have since realized made us resemble cartoon hippos; once we saw pictures. She wore well-scuffed black jazz shoes, which far surpassed my hard white ones in excellence, and I couldn't help but look at them longingly in each class. Her shoes just seemed so pliable, so used, obviously the true sign of a great dancer. And the ratty gray sweatshirt with the neck cut out, Flashdance style, only added to her dance perfection.

My dance clothes paled in comparison. They were cute, I made sure of that; but just too new. Real dancers had holes in their tights; the opposite of my spotless black leotards with cutesy ballet slippers painted just so on the hip. Real dancers had leg warmers that looked dirty, from grand sliding splits across the floor. My leg warmers blinded with bright pink, the color of Pepto-Bismol or thoroughly chewed Hubba Bubba gum, and inexplicably had a royal blue monkey embroidered on them. There's no way I would ever make the Rockettes with attire like that! At this point in my innocent youth, my main cares revolved around my passion for dance and the desire to perform in spangles and heels at Radio City Music Hall. My perspective would soon begin to change.

"My dears," Miss Prudence sighed and let her head fall forward dramatically. Uh oh. We better brace ourselves. She only started sentences with sweet endearments when she wanted to tear into us like a mountain lion. I could see the amber glint of fire in her eye building as her voice stayed calm and yet so menacing. She would eat her prey for sure this time. If only I'd flexed and pointed my feet properly when she'd asked me to. "It hurts my SOUL that you will not even TRY to make these moves work. The song is called, 'In the Mood', and all I see is a bunch of SLOTHS in the mood to look like," she trailed off, clearly on the verge of some dancerly obscenity, then raised her hand, pressed her lips firmly together, and shook her head. She wouldn't let us make her stoop to such degrading levels. Instead, she took a deep breath, steeling herself for more disappointment and pointed to Kirk to give it one last shot before admitting that she'd failed; both herself and her talentless students.

Cue the music.

We pulled our nine-year-old bodies to attention, some better than others. Let's face it, some girls had better builds for dancing than others, and yet it seemed that all girls my age participated, regardless of natural ability. Courtenay, with the lithe body and graceful swan neck and apparently limitless ability to memorize dances in a day, tore up the floor. Eugenia (what a name for a small girl; well, she wasn't that small), clunked around, thrashing her arms as if bushwacking her way through the Amazon, faithfully missing the same steps on every practice run. Nice girl, though. Just should've taken up something a little more well-suited to her natural gifts, whatever those might have been. I fell somewhere in the middle with my talents. I could keep a beat, learn the moves in a moderate amount of time, but I would never dance the superstar solo. The school wouldn't be calling me up to invite me to join the elite Company. Oh how I wished I could join the Company. Instead, stuck with the masses, I tried and toiled and did everything possible to avoid Miss Prudence's Disney villain wrath.

The music swelled. I started to dance, aware of Kirk's reminder gestures through the whole routine. My finger sprung up in a point-and-wiggle just a smidge after his, while I tried to keep time, doing my very best Charleston. *"It didn't take me long to say I'm in the mood, yeah,"* sang the record. And backward walk, kick, ball-change, fanning jazz hands (lots of jazz hands in this routine), and pause, one, two; bouncing to the rhythm before the grand finale. Kirk bounced right along with us, a boat in the waves before a storm, a hopeful look on his face. Could we do it? Could we spin around in unison and land in a half split, again in unison? I had my money on no. I'd seen my parents gamble on a cruise once, so I knew about gambling and odds. But a tiny miracle occurred that day in that small studio. Maybe the cat on Kirk's sweatshirt gave us some sort of "nine lives" inspiration. Somehow all twelve of us rounded our own clumsy feet, looking over our shoulders sassily to the mirror/soon-to-be audience, and we nailed it. As we sat in our half splits, arms in the air in a victory V with fingers splayed wide, our chests heaving with exertion, Kirk began a slow clap straight out of the movies. Miss Prudence, apparently lost in shock, finally noticed his clapping and joined in. They picked up the pace, gestured to us and we began clapping, too. We clapped faster into a frenzy until all of us jumped up from the ground and hugged and squealed as only little girls excel at doing.

Unwilling to break the magic, Miss Prudence quickly, and yet light as air, ran over to the closet in the studio and whisked out a box that held our coveted costumes for the recital. This qualified as the most exciting moment for a young dance student. The arrival of the costume made the routine feel real. With their silver and gold metallics, or lace or satin, and of course, always with their sequins, sequins, and more sequins, dance recital costumes topped all other attire in young girlhood; the crème de la crème of outfits. They made you feel like a movie star, or a princess or an Olympic figure skater, all while making you look like a three dollar hooker; or in our eyes, a grown-up. But we didn't know that at the time, of course. They were amazing; the kind of thing you would wear not just to the recital, but also for Halloween, or putting on shows for family and friends; a parent's favorite event. Very practical. I would argue even more practical than a bridesmaid dress. We DID actually wear them again after the big event. Again and again.

Our "In the Mood" costumes this year did not disappoint. White, with gold and silver metallic. Lace, short tiny skirt, puffy sleeves. I take it back; make that a two dollar hooker. We collectively inhaled sharply, taking in the sparkling majesty of it all, as we tore through the packaging like wrapping paper on Christmas morning. I brought the fabric up to my face and rubbed it against my cheek. Eugenia caught me. I cleared my throat, trying to cover up my indiscretion by quickly rummaging through the empty plastic. I obviously needed to hone my cover-up skills. They would improve with age and experience.

"Okay girls," Miss Prudence said, hanging her adult version of the costume on a nearby hanger. For some reason, Miss Prudence wanted the audience to recognize her as the instructor for the numbers put on by her students, as opposed to those put on by the other instructors in the studio. She accomplished this by wearing an identical matching costume of her own. She was the only one of the instructors to do so. "I need you to do EXACTLY what you just did here in the recital Saturday night. I know you can do it." She didn't look certain. "I know you can." It felt almost like a warning, but the best I think she could do in the form of a pep talk. Kirk stepped forward for a few inspirational words as well.

"I can't believe what I just saw here today, girls." And I couldn't believe what I saw now. Kirk, actually wiping a small tear away. The beauty of our dancing had brought him to tears. Maybe I had a future in dance yet. "I really didn't think you could do it," he said, sniffing. Okay, not really the motivating speech I hoped for, but oh well. "But you managed to put everything you had into the ending and I'll be so proud to see you do it again on that stage. I send you home now with just one thought." We all waited breathlessly. "Don't screw it up." We deflated. No pressure. And should he really say "screw" in front of children? I mean, my dad said it all the time, and worse, but still. As we got up to leave, wrestling with our over-sized plastic garment bags, he motioned for me to stay behind. "Kat, just a sec, please?" Me? Why would he need to single me out?

"I just want to make sure you smile the whole time. You look a little strained. Kinda like you're gritting your teeth or something. Are you in pain?"

"Uh, no," I said, nervous and confused. "Just trying to smile the whole time like you told us to." I didn't think I was in pain.

"Hmm. Okay. Well, try to work on that at home."

"Smiling?"

"Yeah, you know." He pinched the bridge of his nose. I exasperated him so. "Try to make it seem more natural. No more grimacing."

"Okay," I said, dumbfounded. My stage smile looked like a grimace? I thought old people grimaced. Did I look like an old lady? I was only nine. I certainly didn't want anyone confusing me with an old lady. I would definitely have to practice smiling. I hurriedly grabbed my stuff and rustled out the door, trying to hide the red shame inching out of my leotard and up my neck. I didn't want to look like I was in pain. If only I knew what was about to happen.

The Saturday night recital arrived and my nerves had taken hold of me backstage, strangling the glitter out of my spirits. I'd already torn three pairs of panty hose with my irregularly shaped child's nails. At least I'd avoided wearing my very chic Lee Press-Ons; my mother didn't let me leave the house in those. I didn't mind tearing one pair of hose because they ended up having that darker part on top that makes them look like revealing, but not sexy, bike shorts. Or that you just tan weirdly. In the trash with those. I felt a little too young to need control-top, anyway. I finally shimmied, in slow motion, so as not to snag this fourth pair with my costume embellishments, into the lace attire, just in time to see and hear Eugenia throw up all over the floor in her private corner of the room. While Courtenay, and her perfectly svelte physique, felt comfortable stripping down and parading in the middle of the room, girls like Eugenia opted for the intimacy of a corner spot with her back facing out, changing at lightning speed, or as fast as she could go, to avoid any eyes witnessing her perceived lack of body splendor. When my senses got wind of her vomit, I silently rejoiced that she had remained demure. I already had a sensitive stomach and corners are easier to avoid. I could already picture the chain reaction of group vomiting, like a domino display with an olfactory bonus. I tried to divert my attention to get my mind off Eugenia's spew.

My mom hurried into the room to find me after a quick trip to the drug store to pick up blue eyeshadow. She'd had no idea of its necessity. She'd made up my face to look flattering, posh and slightly adult but not overbearing. How stupid of her. She soon realized her mistake once she saw the other girls and their masks of bold color and high gloss. I shuddered, mortified over my overly conservative appearance and sent her post haste to purchase some remedies, preferably in an ocean blue shade. She succeeded in her mission and soon tarted me up like the best girls. My confidence slowly built. She kissed me goodbye and gave me a hug like I might leave for a long journey, which I guess held some truth. A journey into art. I felt powerful.

"Break a leg," she whispered. I felt my power wane. Seeing my furrowed brow, she said, "That means 'good luck' for a person of the stage." A person of the stage. Now I flew back on top of the world, with a much greater angelic wingspan. Go Mom. She blew a kiss as she walked out of the room and the other moms followed suit, fluffing and fixing their daughters one last time as they headed out. Courtenay's mom kept almost making it out the door before having to make one last adjustment. Courtenay just stood there with her arms folded; rolling her eyes, clearly used to what was either her mother's obsessiveness, or caring. You pick.

We heard loud clapping as a number finished up and Miss Prudence rushed back to our room, still in a grotesque red frock with orange ribbon; her matching adult costume for another group. That poor group. They hadn't hit the costume jackpot like we had. Her face shiny, she hurriedly slid out of her ensemble. Without snagging her hose, I noticed. Maybe the sweat made it easier. Within seconds she donned white lace like the rest of us. She applied a fresh coat of red lipstick and voila, she could've been a twin to any of us. A much older twin. A twin of the future.

"This is it, girls," she said in breathless anticipation. "We're up next. Let's kick some, um, tail feathers." We all looked at each other. We were young but not stupid. It's not like we didn't know what word she wanted to say. She always stood on the verge of a bad word. I often wondered if it decreased the badness to use a substitute word when everyone knew the intended word. It seemed like the same thing to me. But I didn't spend this time dwelling on semantics. We had a routine to conquer and I, for one, felt ready to show my skills to the world.

I envisioned critics in the audience, there to write a review somewhere, though I'd never heard of a local dance recital getting press coverage. In my head, a critic appeared as a stodgy old man with a mustache and European accent. He would write, and I would hear the accent in my head, "Well the group was all just mediocre, but there was one standout; a young ingénue, named Kat, who stole the spotlight. Her feet flexed and pointed beautifully at all the right times. And such graceful arm motions. I can't even begin to describe the gorgeous display of her jazz hands. Like fireworks in human form." And so on. I understood the reality, though; an audience comprised of mostly parents, some grandparents, and fidgety siblings, all trying to get comfortable in impossibly uncomfortable folding chairs. The makeup of the audience really made no difference to me. I was an entertainer. I would bring them to their feet. I aimed for nothing less than a standing ovation.

The lighting darkened as we made our way out onto the stage in a straight line, our white lace costumes making us look like participants in some miniature Las Vegas bridal ritual. I could hear a cough, a throat clearing and a couple of whispers emanating from the audience. We would start with our backs to the audience, heads down, for dramatic effect. Hold on. Before I could put my head in the start position, I noticed the back of the stage. Make that the back half of the stage. Five enormous signs, monoliths really, spelling D-A-N-C-E, stood in a semi-circle. So huge that instead of looking down, as assigned, for the routine, I looked up to see the "C" in front of me. It loomed like a plywood Stonehenge. What on earth? They didn't tell us these would decorate the stage. They could have brought this up in rehearsal. I took a deep breath, did a mental "shake it out" and decided that it didn't matter. It's not like this routine involved any stunts or anything.

The music started and I plastered the most un-grimacelike smile I could muster on my face. "In the Mood" had an infectious quality. The audience started tapping their toes. At least, I imagined they did. How could they not? I felt the "boogie" that Kirk kept telling us we needed to embrace to make the routine come to life. I channeled my inner Glenn Miller and felt myself starting to loosen.

My hips swiveled more than they probably should've, my pointer finger wiggled fiercely and with determined rigidity and I smiled, not like an old lady. I had worked long hours on that in the mirror, although I still never really saw what Kirk apparently viewed in my expression. I mean, I don't mind criticism, but come on, give me something I can really work with to make improvements. No matter. Tonight I lit the stage on fire. I might even be, dare I say, Company worthy.

The grand finale approached. We finished up a modest, if not entirely in sync, kick line then broke the line apart, one half of the girls walking/dancing backwards to stage left, the other half towards stage right. I knew only the last few seconds remained before the mind-blowing half-split finish so I wanted to make it count. I threw my whole body, personality, and facial expression repertoire into making my performance memorable. I might've even winked with my mouth opened in a huge "entertainer" smile. Wow, I didn't even know I could wink. During my travels backward, I kept my eyes and grin on the audience and didn't notice Eugenia, the only dancer behind me, in my peripheral vision moving slightly towards the front of the stage. Then I couldn't help but notice. Within a split second, my enthusiastically moving legs flew up above my head as I tumbled rapidly over the sadistically giant letter "E." Dance had tripped me up and made a fool of me. Literally. How did Eugenia know the sign lingered behind her, and how did she know it soon enough to get out of the way? More importantly, why didn't she warn me? A whisper or a darting of the eyes, something. Instead she let me float on down the river and over the waterfall. Tumbling and rolling and banging over the boulders. In the moment, I didn't think these things. I only thought about Miss Prudence's certainly horrified, but resigned, face, and Kirk's frustrated forehead pinching, and most importantly, my mom's words of encouragement.

I leaped up from the sign wreckage, which mostly entailed just me, as the sign stood so large it could've withstood a collision with a Mack truck. But when I returned to my feet, the sudden upright jerk caused the room to go black. I could hear the music, but couldn't see anything. Pure velvety darkness. I panicked and my heart raced. I didn't just "break a leg", I actually broke my head. Or my eyes. Or something. So what did I do at this point? I smiled. Smiled to the point that every one of my teeth must have been showing simultaneously. I kept dancing. There weren't many moves left, but I did them with gusto, even though I couldn't see. Seeing hadn't helped to keep me from falling before, so this couldn't make things much worse. As I danced, the midnight curtain over my vision parted and while hazy at first, I started to see again. The sassy over-the-shoulder look probably didn't come across as I hoped, but at this point I just wanted to land in the half-split at around the same time as everyone else; to redeem myself. We hit the floor. I had tears streaming an overabundance of mascara down my face. I must have looked like a horror movie victim. Carrie with the pig's blood. I might have even cascaded blood, myself. Did mascara just get into my mouth? I still smiled, past the point of performance. I guess I could stop that anytime. Except, I couldn't stop. My mouth was stuck. When I broke my head, I had paralyzed my facial muscles into this performance mask.

Miss Prudence ushered us off the stage to higher applause than I knew we deserved or was even necessary for normal sympathy. Still smiling, I came face-to-face with my mother. She had scurried backstage to greet/rescue me once we returned to the haven of the changing room.

"Baby, are you okay?" she said, sounding more worried than I would've liked. "You did great, you know. That was amazing how you just picked yourself back up and kept going. Perfect." I couldn't respond at first. "That's exactly what you're supposed to do if you fall." She stroked my stiff, shellacked hair and brushed her hand down to rest on my shoulder, lovingly.

"Mom," I said, still smiling broadly. "I think I'm dying."

The VCR sounded like a rapid chipmunk conversation as my parents rewound the tape to show our friends. I worried, actually more like hoped, that the tape would break, seeing as how we'd watched this same piece of it over and over, ad nauseum. And yet, the laughter never seemed to diminish.

"Look! Look! Here it is. Watch closely. Whoops! Right over that letter E," said my father, turning to laugh with the rest of the group; family, friends, some stranger walking his dog outside. I mean really, was my public humiliation that funny? As I listened to the merriment and obligatory, "Ah, poor thing"s, I started to get the idea that this may be the funniest happening in the history of man. Or at least since the invention of dance recitals. I couldn't have chartered new territory by falling on stage. Could I? Well I certainly didn't find it funny at all. And because of my mortification, I entered a new dance school immediately. Life throws enough curve balls without that much shame for an after school activity. I knew that much already. And I wanted the chance to learn from a studio professional enough to understand that you don't include letter towers on the stage with a bunch of nervous, dancing children. I mean, really, what was the purpose of spelling out "DANCE" anyway? Did people not understand that they sat in attendance at a dance recital?

*"Hey Marge, what are all these girls doing on the stage? Are they pretending to be monkeys?"*

*"No dear, look at the sign. They're dancing."*

*"Oh, DANCING! I never would have guessed. I'm sure glad those signs spelled it out for us."*

I felt annoyed. But encouraged. I had heard great things about my new artistic home, the Dance Academy. My best friend, Belle, went there, so that sold me in making the quick change of venues. I needed a fresh start.

Meanwhile, it had taken quite a lot of convincing on my mother's part to make me believe that I had not, indeed, broken my head. But why would I just black out like that?

"Because your adrenaline was up. You got up too fast and the blood rushed to your head."

"But then, if there was a lot of blood in my head, then why was it all black and not, say, red?

"It doesn't work that way, sweetie. It's about blood pressure changes and stuff. It can make you black out. Trust me.

"But…"

"Trust me."

And for the time being I decided to trust her. At that point, I had no reason not to. It wouldn't take long for that to change. But I was young and my mom seemed to know a great deal about everything. I had to believe my parents when they told me everything would be okay. They existed simply to protect me. Besides, I seemed to see fine now; nothing hurt or permanently damaged. I didn't even shed any blood, no thanks to that blasted Eugenia; although she did seem slightly remorseful later on backstage when she acknowledged letting me fall like that. She even threw up one more time for good measure. I only had a small bruise on my tail bone from coming down so hard on it when my feet soared skyward. I thanked the heavens for the silver satin bloomers worn under my costume. At least I didn't bare underwear for the world to witness. Or in my case today, the large group in my living room.

"Let's see it one more time, Dave," said the dog walker to my dad. "It's hilarious." More rapid chipmunk conversation. I went to my room.

\*\*\*

The Dance Academy really upped my game. I no longer agonized about the points and flexes. They started to come to me naturally. How about that? The two sisters, one extremely nice and well-liked, the other militaristic (a former drill sergeant) and mean, who ran the studio were the real deal, not just Olivia Newton John wannabes. They both had trained professionally, both wore highly used, torn up dance attire, and, strangely, both wore three inch false eyelashes. I'm pretty sure the eyelash choice was an offshoot of having performed in Cabaret, but if not, then I could never make heads or tails of that particular embellishment. It certainly made eye contact intense. Heated stare-downs with the Mean One always went her way.

In this forum of dance arts, I found inspiration to experiment with other genres, including a Broadway class called Musical Comedy. Now, I'm no singer. In fact, you don't ever want to hear me even attempt to sing. It puts people off, makes dinner settle not quite right. But in musical comedy class, we all sang and danced, belting it out like actual members of *A Chorus Line*. And in a group setting, I didn't sound that bad. My off key voice blended quite well with the others who had more talent and it made something that sounded almost melodic and entertaining.

After a year in the Dance Academy, more haughty and intelligent than my old school, The Dance Zone, I knew that falling over letter "E" signs could fade into my past. I had turned ten now and grown wiser; more mature. I no longer wore my monkey leg warmers. I had endured the Mean One's verbal barbs, and turned her criticisms of my form into positive changes. She would walk around the room banging a large metal rod to the beat of the music while we did our floor stretches. If she happened to catch an appendage with the rod, so be it. You should've known better than lay in her way. You learn fast to improve, if you fear pain. Trust me. I'd already started cultivating this fear. I performed like the Pavlov's dog of dancers. As a reward, I would participate in four routines this year, instead of the paltry one that I had demolished last year.

*** 

The weekend of the recital came around and I could tell at home that my parents' nervousness for me had skyrocketed. While they'd found almost unimaginable joy in sharing the video of my previous collapse with the universe, they did worry about my well-being and hoped that I wouldn't reach the same fate again. They were decent people after all. Maybe they had joked so much about the fall as a defense mechanism to mask the real agony they felt on my behalf. Like clowns. I smiled frequently at them, to ease their suffering, and repeatedly assured them that I wouldn't break my head this time.

"But you didn't break your head before," my mother said.

I held up my hand. Not the point. I think a little of the drama of dance had started to rub off on me. Or maybe I just missed Kirk and Miss Prudence a little. Maybe I should start talking with exaggerated emphasis. My SOUL stands on the line, so I must TRY to FEEL the music coursing through my BODY. I believed nothing would go wrong. Or could go wrong. I'd already had my time of wrong. How naïve.

I scratched my neck as I watched my mom shrug and go back to making lunch. We would only have a few hours after lunch to relax, and for me to practice before the show; so we tried to get everything together to avoid feeling rushed at the last minute. I scratched the other side of my neck. Did a mosquito get in here?

I went into the bathroom to look at my neck. What the…? I had four or five bumps on my neck, but noticed that one half-peeked out of the neck ring of my tee shirt; still the shirt I'd slept in and hadn't changed out of. Don't judge. I wasn't trying to be lazy. Just hadn't gotten around to changing by lunchtime.

I lifted up my shirt and revealed an extremely red, bumpy, covered pale belly and screamed.

"MOM! GET IN HERE! NOW!"

I started heaving, mostly because I was grossed out by the pizza on my torso, but also because as soon as I saw it, I combined the view of the bumps with the feeling on my neck and everything started itching at once. I lowered the shirt and used it to rub my stomach manically, rather than scratching with my nails.

"What? What is it?" she said. She spoke calmly, probably used to the histrionics of young girls by now, rarely involving anything actually serious.

I squeezed my eyes together and gently, slowly lifted my shirt up so she could see. I heard her gasp and opened my eyes quickly. That wasn't what I wanted to hear.

"What's wrong with me?" I asked.

"Well," she turned me towards the light so she could get a better view. "Have you been around anyone with chicken pox lately?"

"Chicken pox? NO!" I looked at her frantically. "Is that what this is? You think I have chicken pox? I CAN'T have chicken pox. I have a recital in..," I looked at my watch for effect, even though I didn't wear a watch in those days; not until Swatches came out a year or so later, "like FIVE hours!"

"Shh. Okay. Look, calm down." She stood back and put her hands on her hips, thinking mode. "I'll call the doctor. And I think I have some calamine lotion. Just sit tight." Okay, she would fix this. Not the end of the world. Besides, after tonight, it didn't matter if I had chicken pox. Just get through tonight and all will return to normal. It's not like they existed all over me. I scratched behind my ear. Great.

She came back in five minutes later with a crusty looking bottle of pink potion and a renewed sense of purpose.

"I'm going to put this on you. It'll feel cool and hopefully make it stop itching. I'm going to run up to the store to get you an oatmeal bath. The doctor said it'll soothe your skin. He said you couldn't perform tonight and here are some socks to put over your hands to keep you from scratching." She softly but swiftly rubbed the lotion in circles on all the affected areas. It really felt good on the itching.

"Wait, what?" I asked, just now hearing everything she'd said. "I can't perform?" My voice cracked and large tears formed in my eyes, my lips malformed from an annoying twitch.

"Well that's what he said, but here's what I'm thinking," she said, looked directly at me, hopeful. "I think we calm the itch, keep you cool and relaxed and you do your show tonight. It's only a few dances. And you've worked so hard. I'd hate for you to miss them. I'll call your instructors and tell them what's going on. You may have to be in some sort of quarantine backstage so other girls won't catch it, 'cause you're probably really contagious, but you could still dance." Contagious? Oh my god, I'm a pariah! A leper! How disgusting. People will talk about this for ages. The girl who can't get through one recital without falling or being forced into quarantine with an infectious disease. Fantastic. My mother pulled me out of my self-loathing with these words:

"I can't believe you have chicken pox. Jimmy's dad got them and they turned into Shingles and he was in so much pain and had to go to the hospital for two weeks. He missed so much work." I just stared at her with saucer eyes. Why did she tell me this? Holy cow. What were shingles? And when would my itching pox turn into these painful, flaky, blistering boils of melting skin?

"Okay, there you go. All covered. Now go rest up and try not to get yourself into too much of a state over any of this. You'll feel better." I just kept staring at her, dumbfounded.

I managed to stay cool and not to scratch myself too often, although let's face it, I cheated a little. Maybe a couple of bumps developed a dual quality of itching and pain from the scratching. And even though entirely self-inflicted by my nails, I may have focused too much on this developing pain and what it might indicate. I could tell the shingles were forming and multiplying, like Gremlins with food and water. But we packed up and headed to the performance auditorium. I would not let my illness beat me. I'd worked too hard.

Luckily my favorite performance came first. Musical Comedy. We performed from no less than Cabaret. Maybe the sisters subconsciously wanted us to all don three inch eyelashes as well, although the ratio of lash length to our height would have made for something truly special. We would perform "Money (makes the world go around)", and I'd already affixed my gold beret with the gold sequined dollar sign to the only part of my body that didn't itch; my hair. I pulled on my solid gold leotard and mini skirt over my bumps. I seriously felt like a Solid Gold Dancer and I loved it. The fabric, a rough metallic material, looked and felt like Brillo pad. It worked perfectly, as it continually scratched every itch, scrubbing my skin like the dirtiest of dishes. Nobody could accuse me of cheating now. My nails ventured nowhere near my skin. I'd already learned the fine art of loopholes years before law school. My mother had tried to help me clean all the pink of the dried lotion off, but it had made me itch more, so I had a psychedelic leopard quality to me as I took the stage. A virtual pink panther, glimmering with pink and gold like a New Jersey housewife.

The dance started in the dark; they usually do to provide an element of "Ahhh" as the lights come up and the music starts. The lights popped just as "Money" blared and boy did they emit a lot of heat. I immediately started sweating, and the sweat trickled under the Brillo fabric and the itching soon followed. I couldn't control myself. I swooped around and before I shot my arm out in unison with the other girls, I briefly detoured my hand across my stomach for a quick scratch. You wouldn't notice if you weren't paying very close attention; it was that fast. When we turned our back to the audience and proceeded to go down the line, almost wave-style with our arms reaching up straight, I managed to scrape my hands, very subtly up and down my neck. *"Money, money, money. Money money money. Money money money, oooooh."* Ooooh, was right. I punctuated every move with a scratch until that became my main dance step. I'd inadvertently taken the solo I so often craved. At least I scratched to the beat of the music and emoted with all my might. We finished and I ran off the stage feverishly attacking all of the skin on my torso.

Once again my mother met me backstage. I had a feeling I'd created another showstopper they could share with the masses; a video masterpiece. Instead, she carried remorse in her eyes and she just shook her head when she saw me.

"I'm such a terrible mother. I can't believe that I sent you out there like that. I'm so sorry." She took this moment to worry about her parenting skills. How selfish.

"Mom, don't worry about that," I said. I had more important matters to discuss than my embarrassing, and repeated, dance failures or my mother's supposed "stage mother" tendencies. "I think my chicken pox have turned into shingles. You better get me to the hospital."

She stared at me, saw my seriousness, and just started to laugh.

Hypochondriac Lesson #2:
Be rational. Or, in the alternative, talk to someone rational.

*2- Vaseline Anyone?*

In the year 1987, I turned twelve years old. Big hair dominated the style scene and mine was accordingly large and full of unruly attitude; like an adult's huge lioness mane had been superimposed on a regular child's body. Too bad I didn't have a firm grasp on how to tame or manage it properly. See, I have very thick, jet fuel colored, naturally curly hair. How thick? Well, so thick that every time I've ever gone to any hair salon to have it cut, and I mean every time, the beautician will say, "Wow! You have really thick hair. Did you know that?" And she'll pull and tug in vain with a comb at the knots. Nope, never heard that before. It's not like I've broken that many brush handles on it or anything. Glad you were there to point it out, lady. Add my uncooperative coif to my caterpillar-like eyebrows (or as I preferred to think of them, Brooke Shieldsian), and figure in my awkwardly changing adolescent body and you can clearly understand why I thought 1987 the perfect year to enter a beauty pageant.

I know what you must think. Between the dancing bit and now the beauty pageant, you think my mother really thrived as an overbearing talent mom and forced me into such sordid affairs. While I agree that beauty pageant contestants often have lunatic parents, I have to admit that the idea for the pageant belonged completely to me. For some reason, words like "poise" and "grace" and "prizes" started to carry importance to me. I don't know why. But I wasn't ready for boys yet, so I decided to focus my attention elsewhere. My parents knew the mayor of our town, a personal friend, and he just happened to have a young wife (second or third wife); an ex-beauty queen. She agreed to train me. Oh yes, walking out on that stage, making a few turns and hopefully advancing far enough to have the opportunity to answer a bland question about current affairs or my personal ambitions requires much training. I flutter with joy, and a slight stomach ache, just thinking about it now.

Technically, I'd already had my first foray into pageantry. A couple of years back I'd entered into a contest at the local mall. I'm not sure why anyone thought parading dolled-up children on a stage at a mall was a good idea; seems like catnip for pedophiles to me, and only adds to the number of strangers that will bear witness to your humiliation if you mess up something. I didn't win. Or even come close. It's pretty much standard practice that the first time you enter one of these things you move around on stage as a complete outsider. They take your entrance fee money, probably laugh at you, and continue laughing as they deposit it in the bank. I didn't stun anyone as a ten-year-old in a large, ruffly, teal green dress with Bea Arthur hair. To illustrate just how out of touch I was with the process, I actually listed my mom's teriyaki chicken as my favorite food. For the record, the correct answer is pizza. Now I understood the skills I needed to possess and eagerly used the professional at my disposal. I felt like an insider with the upper hand; like I had the support of the pageant mob.

I met twice with Ex-Beauty Queen and she whipped me right into shape. It all happened like a montage scene and if there'd been a song accompanying the changes, it would've been something like, *"She's the best girl, but you wouldn't have know it under all that hair. She's the best girl, she's now so pretty, she'll no longer scare."* Or something to that effect. Cut me some slack. I'd only begun my bad poetry phase, so song lyrics may have suffered from lack of experience. Anyway, the first episode of the montage included the maiden voyage of tweezers into my sea of eyebrows. More accurately, eyebrow. Ex-Beauty Queen came at me with a pair, like a butcher attacking a fresh cut of meat, but I soon saw the furrow in her own perfect arches, and we quickly hopped in the car and headed to get them waxed. There's only so much one lady with a single set of tweezers could do. And we didn't want her worried wrinkles to turn permanent.

Next, we tackled the "Looking." When you walk out on stage, you can't just smile. You might as well wear a neon sign that says "Amateur." You must have points where you direct your eyes around the room. But, the trick is to hit all these points without looking like you're trying to hit all these points; straight ahead, then down to the judges, gliding your head along the row of them, bobble head style. Then up, (look there's the audience, hi) and over the top of what you can't see because the bright, hot lights will blind your eyes. Then always eye contact again with the judges to finish it off and make them realize you have the goods and deserve all accolades; most importantly that sash and, hold me down, that coveted crown.

The "Walking" comprised the final piece of the ugly duckling-into-swan montage. That cool 80's guitar/synthesizer music has been playing this whole time, in case you forgot. At this point, the music in my head swelled and turned even more inspirational; the Chariots of Fire moment. Even though my dress would puff out to eternity, late nineteenth century southern belle style, I had to make sure my feet made no mistakes. Like the Looking, the Walking isn't just walking; you certainly can't merely walk out, turn and walk back. You might as well admit you've just crawled from under the nearest rock at that rate. There's an elegance and a routine. Walk, stop, Look (at all agreed upon points), turn, stop, look over your shoulder (pretty much you are showing off your rear-end), THEN, you get to walk back to the line or off stage. It holds so many more complexities than the credit it receives; it's the advanced math version of walking. Ex-Beauty Queen did her very best with me. Now I held the burden to carry it off without a stumbling tragedy. That, apparently, was a tall order.

Three days before the pageant, I started my period. And I mean started, for the very first time ever in my life. I knew a little about it, in the sense that I knew it would happen once a month for much of my life, knew that it would last a few days each time, knew that my mother usually stayed in a fairly bad mood when having hers, and knew it meant that I would bleed. I thought I knew it all. Unfortunately, I'd missed the all-important "boys in one room, girls in the other" discussion during the fifth grade. Let this be a warning against allowing your kids to stay home from school. My parents either forgot or didn't think they needed to sit down with me to have a conversation. I don't really know what happened, but we had a definite lack of communication on that subject because when it commenced, I had no idea what to do. What is THAT? In hindsight, it seems crazy that I would be confused, but back then, I grew so terrified that I started kneeling by my bed on the hour to pray that I wouldn't die.

For starters, I didn't have any cramps. Nothing. Just suddenly, something. And it didn't appear red, like any other blood I'd seen in my entire life. Instead it came out, gag (sorry to be gross), brown. The Internet did not yet exist on which to look this up and the 1952 encyclopedia set we had, which I used for all of my papers in school - the entry for "computer" was just a few short sentences; I was very current- did not provide any quality information to address my concerns. I had reached the end. I felt sure of it. Each year after Christmas, I would say a prayer that my parents and I would live at least until the following Christmas. How's that for a youthful hypochondriac? But this time, God seemed not to have answered my prayer. An only child and my parents would lose me so young. I couldn't tell them. It would just break their hearts. Not entirely clear on anatomy at the time - I was only absent that one day from school, yet I missed so much- and too fearful to do much exploring, I couldn't properly diagnose the exact source of the problem. But I knew it was serious. You just don't emit some sort of non-blood fluid unless you have something fatal. So I folded up some toilet paper and put it in my underwear and tried to pretend that my life would not end in the foreseeable future. A true beauty queen rises above all adversaries, and that includes the Grim Reaper.

The day of the pageant, I found myself still in the throes of death. I'd stayed mostly quiet for the week, and I think my parents chalked it up to nerves. Oh how they would cry when they learned the sad, horrible truth. I hoped they would pick a picture of me for the funeral with my hair looking decent. We packed up my outfits for the contest; interview outfit-so that a bunch of twelve-year-old girls could wear shoulder pads and look like office drones; the spunky pageant t-shirt and red shorts for our initial stage parade; and of course, the pièce de resistance, the ball gown, and headed towards the airport Holiday Inn ballroom. The organizers really pull out all the stops for these events. They provide nothing but the best and an overwhelming air of classiness. And Aquanet hairspray.

"Welcome to the Tenth Annual Little Miss United States Florida Pageant," said the MC, in a deep, powerful voice like a wrestling match announcer. "The event we've all been waiting for." Did he really say that out loud? Did he mean it as a joke? Aside from the fear of my impending death, I'd been pretty excited about it, but I wondered if the audience had also waited for the day of the pageant with baited breath. I looked around the room to gauge the reaction from the other girls and mothers, but the girls all had their game faces on and the mothers concentrated heavily, deeply engrossed in grooming and preening their offspring, these smaller versions of themselves who now bore the burden of their dreams of greatness.

A petite diva, whose body looked about ten, but whose head looked about thirty-six, pushed her mother's hand away as it came at her face with more powder.

"Enough, Mommy," she said. "Daddy said not to let you make me look like a prostitute." The mother flinched and looked frantically around her to make sure nobody had heard. I looked up at my mother who bit her lip to keep from laughing and didn't make eye contact.

"Do you even know what that word means?" asked the diva's mother. The diva shook her head yes, confidently. "I know your father certainly does," the mother added under her breath.

"Yes, Mommy, a prostitute is a lady who wears too much makeup and doesn't know her manners. She chews gum in public and wears tight clothes." My mother inadvertently let a noise escape from her lips. The diva's mother heard her and immediately ushered the diva to the other side of the room to regain composure and complete the primping process.

My mother looked down at me, her expression asking, "Am I doing the right thing here?"

"How're you feeling, sweetie?" she asked, smoothing down my pageant tee shirt.

I touched her hand. I had to put her at ease about her mothering skills. I mean she WAS about to lose her only child to a mysterious illness.

"I'm great. Why don't we get you some water or a snack?" The child becomes the parent. She reluctantly agreed.

As we turned to walk over to a refreshment station, a hairbrush sailed through the air, having missed its intended target of a mother's head. We turned in unison to locate the assailant and saw a miniature princess standing next to a hanging dress of layered fuchsia frills. The dress seemed to shrink back from her wrath, just like her mother.

"Mother, I told you. NO RIBBON!" she screamed and stamped each foot in turn, causing her long hair to bounce against the pink taffeta of her dress. "I only want sparkly in my hair. NO RIBBON!" More stomps.

"Oh for Christ's sake, fine. Don't make a big deal out of it. I just want you to look perfect," said the mother, defeated, as if used to the verbal and physical assaults.

"I am perfect, Mommy. I'm going to win. They all know it." She gestured around the room, casting a look of disgust at the collective, then performed a graceful pirouette.

Another little girl, who strongly favored a porcelain china doll, turned to her mother and asked, "Mommy, what's wrong with that little girl? Why is she so mean?" The mother took a long look at the offender and the offender's blanching mother.

"I think she was raised that way." Then she turned back to her own child. "Let's get that smudge off your face. We can't have you going out on stage with a dirty face."

My mom leaned down to my ear. "I'm so glad you're you," she whispered. I think we both experienced a modicum of shock by the spectacle of all the little girls and the candy-colored dresses hanging around the room like colored sprinkles on a bland cupcake.

"Girls, you're up," said a tall brunette woman with well-coiffed hair. The stage director of the competition.

We queued up by number and waited hand-in-hand with our mothers, or handlers, to go on parade for the judges, all wearing our white pageant tees and red shorts. The mothers, eagerly standing next to their charges before sending them off on stage, gave the appearance they were about to run their prize Golden Retrievers around the ring at Westchester. The line inched forward until I reached the curtain.

"Contestant number 12, please take the stage," the tall MC said into the microphone.

I stood rooted to the rough patch of floor, running my foot nervously over the bump made by electrical cords taped down backstage. Why all the tape on the cords? Probably to avoid tangling, or so that people wouldn't trip over them in their finery and cause a scene. I couldn't hear the announcements very well as the speakers stood like sentries, facing the audience. I found myself staring at the blatant comb-over on the MC. Silver and twisty and strange to behold. Did he really think he fooled anybody with that?

"Contestant number 12?"

"Sweetie, you're up," my mom said, gently giving me a shove in my lower back to propel me forward.

I startled and my eyes refocused. I inhaled deeply to calm my nerves. I was ready. Bring it on. I straightened my shoulders, held my head high, just as Ex-Beauty Queen had trained me to do, and started to walk gracefully out onto the stage. I heard a strange noise from behind me that sounded very much like my mother, but I certainly couldn't stop now. The lights blinded me, forcing me to use every ounce of willpower to keep smiling and not raise a hand to shield my eyes. I was the proverbial deer, staring at headlights, or in this case, stage lights, in the middle of the runway. I felt protective tears spring into my ducts, but I would not let myself squint. I couldn't look in pain, even though, boy, this really hurt my eyes. The Vaseline on my teeth, another critical beauty queen trick, made sure my lips didn't stick, but nothing could stop the tremor where my cheeks met my mouth. Muscle fatigue plagued me from smiling too hard. The more I willed the twitching to stop, the more I felt like I might start seizuring all over. Beauty queens did not have seizures!

I thought I heard laughter, but couldn't really tell with each heartbeat swooshing through my ears. The lights burned and I could feel the sweat trickling down my leg. Odd. My armpits, usually the first to sweat, strangely did not perspire. Nor my back. I'm just nervous. Nothing to see here. *"Kat is in the sixth grade. She loves dancing, reading, spending time with friends, and her favorite food is... pizza."* I heard the appreciative response in the audience. I told you I knew the right answer was pizza. The lights warmed me as if I lay under the heat lamp at a restaurant waiting to be served for dinner to the next paying customer. I turned around at the end of the stage, vertical rotisserie style, and attempted to make my way back up the runway. Upbeat children's tunes that had been morphed into elevator music played over the loud speaker. Then a flash. The massive light from a commercial camera aggressively shot brightness at my face. It didn't matter, though; I'd made it without incident out and back over that T-shaped platform that served as the stage for the first phase of the competition. But I certainly needed to freshen up. The itching sweat trickle drove me crazy.

Again, this was becoming a habit with us, my mother met me backstage with an expression that meant something horrible had happened, like an ax murderer on the loose at the Holiday Inn, or food poisoning in the banquet facilities, or a torn dress.

"I think we need to make a quick trip to the bathroom," she said and ushered me away from the changing room so quickly that I didn't even have a chance to ask why.

"What's going on? I have to get into my interview outfit," I said. Didn't she understand we were on a time crunch? Every minute I wasted in here meant that the other divas would have that time to make themselves even more perfect.

"Baby, you've started your period." She looked down, forcing my eyes down with hers. "All over the place."

"Oh my god!" I paused. "Oh. My. God." Then I fell silent. "Wait...wait...," I processed the ramifications. "Do you know what this means?" I asked, growing more excited.

"Well, yeah. We've got a bit of a mess to clean up here. And, I mean, there are some things we should probably talk about."

"NO! I mean, sure, okay. Whatever. I mean, I'm not DYING!" I grabbed her hands into my own and jumped up and down.

"Dying? Why would you think you're dying?"

"Well I've had...stuff...coming out of me for, like, three days now. But I didn't think it was my period because it wasn't red." My mom exhaled audibly and started laughing, a sound so much better than the expected sobs from hearing the news.

"Oh, child of mine. Where do you get such crazy ideas? Next time, instead of sitting on information like this, why don't you just come to me? I'll clear things up for you." She couldn't keep the giggle out of her voice. It wasn't THAT funny. "Now wait here while I go get something for your little problem at the gift shop. I'll be right back."

I stared at myself in the mirror. I would live. I'd been saved. For now. I couldn't help but notice that strange things were happening to me and my body on a more regular basis. But at this moment, I sat on top of the world. When she returned with my "womanly supplies" (because wasn't I officially a woman now?), I became a little woman with a mission. I owned those shoulder pads and tore up the interview competition. Then I donned my beautifully large iridescent pink gown, smoothed down my elegant bob- that had taken a lot of wrangling and hair spray- and blew everyone away. Everyone, that is, except for the four people who beat me. But who cares about little details? I earned fourth runner-up in the Little Miss United States Florida Pageant. I felt so ecstatic I could've screamed but that would've been so unladylike, so I smiled my slick Vaseline smile and waved my princess, screwing-in-a-light-bulb, wave. Today I came close to the grand title of beauty queen. But more importantly, today I would not die. And if all continued to go well, I would fulfill my annual prayer and make it to Christmas again.

Hypochondriac Lesson #3:
Don't make a fool of yourself if you don't have to.

### 3- *Living Every Day Like You Just Made a Hole-in-One*

"A hush falls over the crowd," said the teenager, into the microphone of the PA system, infusing his dramatic tone with teenage sarcasm. "Tim Donnelly's hoping to make this putt, so he can tie up the score. Can he do it? Can he beat the twelve-year-old prodigy?" He turned to my mother, covering the mike, "Even if she's the boss' daughter."

My mother fake smacked him on the arm, something probably hugely punishable under current employment laws. "You better watch it, Mister." She pointed at him in mock anger. "And you better hope Kat didn't hear the twelve bit. She's thirteen now and won't be underestimated." I was actually standing close enough to hear her say this to him, trying not to blush, waiting for Tim Donnelly's final putt. The guy practiced ALL the time. Surely he would make it. Swing, clink, the ball rolled gently and assuredly into the cup. He did a fist pump and let out a loud "Whoop" like he just won the Masters. That's alright, Tim. I let you have that one. I'll get you next time, when it really counts; when there's a trophy involved.

See, I grew up in unique circumstances. While most kids had parents who worked at an office and came home to a nice home-cooked meal each night, living normal lives, I had something entirely different. My parents owned and ran a miniature golf course. Lets Putt America. Grammatically incorrect with no apostrophe, of course. Nobody seemed to notice. Fifty-four putting holes made up the three courses, each designed lovingly by my father. I still remember all his long nights with drafting paper, like an architect designing an important skyscraper. This course didn't have windmills and fake mountains, but encapsulated the look of an authentic golf course, where the green carpet on each hole held well-thought-out obstacles and realistic traps. With practice, you could conquer the holes, unlike lame (but arguably fun) courses with say, a dragon mouth, where players relied entirely on chance as to where the ball would go when struck.

As if that weren't enough, we had a large, looping go-cart track at the back end of the property and a clubhouse which held an arcade and frozen yogurt shop inside its gingerbread façade. My parents let me name the business when I was nine and I came up with the riveting title of Yummy Yogurt with Terrific Toppings. What a life for a young kid. I got to gorge myself on frozen treats all the time. I stayed up late most nights because, unless my mother took me home (which for some reason I will never understand, was rarely), the whole family stayed to close up shop around eleven at night. Then, we might even go someplace cool, like Denny's or Perkins, for pancakes and pie. Rest assured that my definition of a cool restaurant has changed as I've aged. Truth be told, a lot of kids envied me. For a while, anyway.

The business and our life as a family intertwined and turned into one. We spent more time there than we did in our house. Well, why not? More to do. In a suburban part of Orlando, we had developed an entertainment hot spot for the locals, who wanted to enjoy a life outside of tourism. You could either go bowling or come to us, if you wanted to do something besides go to Disney. We knew everybody. Cops, local politicians, business owners, rich people, poor people. It was great. At the moment, I attended middle school and LOVED the fact that all the coolest kids from the high school worked for us. My father made it a practice to hire only the most popular, attractive kids; also an employment practice that would probably not hold up too well today. I felt so mature and special and in-the-know; even though I later found out that the "Boss's Daughter" was by far NOT the worst thing they called me. Whatever; I lived in ignorant bliss. I had a ludicrous crush on the star football player, who was the homecoming king, and a senior. I mean, really? I was in the eighth grade for cryin' out loud. He got so annoyed with me one time that he actually picked me up, took me outside and threw me into the dumpster; the dumpster that we shared with the neighboring shopping center. That we shared with Perkins and Checkers. Gross! Even so, I had stars in my eyes. He was just so cute.

Anyway, that's beside the point. Our little community business became such a staple of entertainment for some people that we decided to do what all good mini-golf establishments should. We started a tournament. We weren't sure anyone would want to take part. I mean bowling alleys offered bowling leagues, but would anyone have interest in mini-golfing on a weekly basis in a competitive way? Some people actually classified bowling as a sport. Athletes played it in the Olympics or something, right? But mini-golf? Not so much. Well pinch my backside and call me Pumpkin. Fifty-six people showed up for our first Wednesday night tournament. And here I thought that our establishment catered mostly to teenage boys bringing girls out on a date. We typically served as the alibi given to the parents. We were just the stop after the fast food joint, but before the boys took the girls someplace to try to score. At least that's how it always seemed to me. But it turns out people truly craved a routine of fun; a day of escape. Our tournaments offered camaraderie, a sense of belonging to something bigger than yourself, and cheese nachos.

After a few weeks, a few regulars, stand-outs really, emerged. There was Tim, my nemesis, a man who dressed entirely in seventies polyester, preferring a palette of burgundy and sky-blue. He took mini-golfing VERY seriously and frequently spoke of his days on a real golf course; nothing quite believable. If his stories could be trusted, then why wasn't he still playing "real" golf, like in the good ol' days? He functioned as my main competition. He tolerated me.

Bachelor number two, Steve, taught math at the local high school, and inappropriately ogled all the hot teenage girls who worked for us, many of them his students. We often asked him if that would get him in trouble. He would shrug and smile. He was in his early thirties and lived with his mother. He always wore school coach-type shorts; colored polyester shorts with high snap waists and a length just north of anything actually in style. Now that I think about it, he may have actually worked as a coach at the high school, but he probably would've worn the shorts anyway. I mean, he didn't coach anyone while he played mini-golf but he still wore them.

Third on the roster was Marvin, a tall, meek, lonely man who just wanted attention. My parents and I bet that he'd probably never had a date in his life. He would later go on to marry a very attractive woman, but he would shake so badly at the altar during the wedding that a groomsman would have to literally hold him up so he could finish his vows. True story. I sat in the pew, nudging my parents ferociously while it happened, hoping they wouldn't miss it. Marvin was one of the nicest men of all time and he and Steve would frequently join us for our late night dinners, and, in a turn of events that was normal then, but seems weird in retrospect, they started visiting our house each week to watch the show *Moonlighting*. Just to watch that show, nothing else.

My favorite, or rather favorite to make fun of in my head (I swear I'm not inherently a mean person, but this guy gave me so much to work with), was a guy named Bob. Bob, approaching his late twenties, did not have a car, so rode his bike everywhere. Great, you say. How cool and environmentally conscious. No, that's not it. He just didn't have the gumption to get a driver's license. But he also didn't really know how to properly ride his bike. He wrecked all the time. So often that he'd worn off some of the large wale corduroy from the shorts he wore every day with his skidding. He didn't wear a helmet and, well, he was a mess. His dark hair parted clearly in the middle, but puffed grotesquely so it looked like he had a butt up there. And he would play golf, lift one leg, bend it at the knee and pass gas. In front of everyone. Didn't even bother acknowledging it. Yeah, Buddy. We heard that. And saw it. And smelled it. Plus, we used to have these clever little suction cups (Putter Cups) that you could attach to the end of your club so that you could use the club to pick up the ball rather than bend over every time. Bob would write a score down and rest his club up against his crotch so that the suction cup allowed some ball to rest gently on it, even though it was NOT the golf ball (Bob ball, if you must know). My parents always tried to teach me to include everyone, but somehow they never invited him to watch *Moonlighting*.

The final figure in our tournament cast of characters was Marco, a Seventh Day Adventist who made his improbably hot wife dress matronly and eat tofu before tofu tasted chic and delicious. He had apparently known my father when my dad ran his dad's miniature golf course in Miami. Yes, the mini-golf lineage in my family goes way back. That's also where my mom and dad met. It was seriously in my blood. I guess that history contributed to us enduring him now. Marco spent any free moments he had with me, grilling me with logic puzzles, laughing directly at me when I couldn't figure them out, and making me feel otherwise uncomfortable. I guess I can credit him with inadvertently helping me do well on the LSAT later on in life; so much of that relies on logic puzzles. At the time, I found his conversations with me creepy and I tried to keep my distance.

Our tournaments built, bracket style, so that by the end of the night, one winner would emerge. We capitalized on the success and decided to create more excitement by designing a try-out for a grand tournament that would have fabulous prizes, and trophies. I was a girl obsessed and made my parents order trophies that had both girl and boy figures on top, just in case. The local radio station would come out, do live broadcasts and give away cruise vacations and other swag; so thrilling to an eighth grader. I couldn't wait and neither could the crowd. The practicing commenced. This was very clever on my dad's part; people would have to spend money to practice at our place as we owned the only mini-golf course around. Can you say monopoly?

Two weeks before the big final tournament, my parents sat me down in our kitchen with the country décor (always a puzzler to me as my dad grew up in high falutin' debutante style, and my mother grew up hillbilly, one of ten kids in Kentucky, but not in a "gingham and cute ducks" country style). My mother and father glanced at each other, as if to confirm that they really wanted to say their next words and looked at me with sympathy eyes. Uh oh. What was wrong with me?

"Kat." Always a bad sign when they started with my name. "Kat," my mother said again, trying to bring herself to utter the next words. "Would you like to know if I find out I have cancer and might die?" Um, what? What the bleep kind of question is that? I never had, nor ever planned to use a cuss word in front of my parents; not even in my head.

"You have cancer?"

"No."

"Then what're we talking about here?"

"Well, your dad and I went to the dermatologist today. He has to have a bunch of pre-cancers taken off his head." She pointed to my dad's bald head, while he leaned over to show me the scabby looking flakes that I just took for granted as natural topography for the follicly challenged. "But I have that red mole on my back and they looked at it today." She paused like she might start crying.

"Yeah?"

"They cut it off because they thought it might be something. A biopsy, they call it. I won't know for a few days. But if it's cancer then, who knows." Wow. Who knows? Those were some words with endless possibilities, most of which I couldn't have even fathomed at the time.

"But it could be okay, right?" I asked, wringing my hands.

"Yeah, of course. We just wanted to find out from you, you know, if it's not okay. Would you want to know?"

"Yes, I would want to know. Are you crazy? You're my mother."

"Okay, fine then. I'll let you know." They got up from the table. End of conversation. I'll let you know. Like, I'll let you know if I can swing by after school. Or, I'll let you know if you can go to the movies with your friends. I'll let you know if you can have ice cream after dinner. Something seemed rather wrong about saying, "Well, I'll let you know if I have cancer." And if my dad had pre-cancers, whatever that really meant, and my mom potentially had cancer, what did that mean for me? I lived in the sun as much as they did.

I slowly rose from the table, meandered back to my bedroom, like any other ordinary day, shut my door, then, in a frenzy, removed my clothes; like some imaginary force had set them on fire. One whole wall of my room contained a mirror with a ballet bar across the center (we didn't install that; it came with the house; a huge selling point for me). I inspected every single freckle on my body. I was fair skinned and I was in the sun every day, so I had LOTS of freckles. Were any of them red? That seemed a problem for the one on my mother. No. No red ones. That one on my shoulder has a weird shape. And look at that one on my stomach. My leg! Oh, my leg had a strange mole! Okay. Calm down. These were all probably fine. Just freckles. But still, they didn't all look uniform. Something

had to be wrong. The whole family could have skin cancer. Was that possible?
It's not contagious, is it? I put my clothes back on, only now fully aware of each
strange spot on my body, each invader, rooted to my skin like a killer fungus. I
would need to make some serious changes if I thought I could survive this plague
of moles.

When the day of the tournament finals arrived, I inwardly cursed my parents
for starting it in the middle of the day. It made perfect sense, in that they needed
to allow enough time to do each round. We couldn't be here all night. But still, a
sunny day in Central Florida created a definite problem for skin cancer survivors
like us. The results came back for my mom. She was clean. They wanted to take
the whole mole out of her back; what they described as a half dollar coin in size.
The doctors just wanted to remain cautious so that it wouldn't turn into anything
later or continue to grow.

My parents dismissively announced the news to me a couple of days after they
found out, and almost as an afterthought.

"Oh, by the way, I don't have cancer. False alarm." Proceed as usual,
apparently. Did they not take into account that they'd terrorized me to my very
core? I couldn't just shake it off. It had been too close of a call for my taste.
They were content to move on with their regular activities and sun worship, but
I developed an obsession with UV ray safety. I had this vision that skin cancer
shriveled you up and maybe even caused part of your skin to fall off. I was young
and trying to look cute. That wouldn't really be possible with a pruny or blackened
epidermis.

I saw no choice but to enter the tournament looking like Michael Jackson;
not the way he looked then as an African American, but the way he looked later
on, like a deranged mental hospital escapee. I had completely slathered myself

in sunblock to the point that a passer-by could rub up against me and then have proper sun protection for the day. I wore a long-sleeved white cotton shirt, long linen pants, sunglasses and a hat with a brim and long flaps hanging off the back in two swaths. I looked like I should ride a camel in the Sahara, not play prize-winning mini-golf in suburban Orlando. It helped (well, depending on your perspective) that my father had adopted the flap hat look as well. He, at least, took the pre-cancer thing somewhat seriously, I guess. Only, he hadn't bothered to purchase a hat with actual attached flaps. Rather, always eager to promote the business, he wore a regular Lets Putt America baseball cap with a hand towel draped over his bald head underneath. Maybe this is how he imagined MacGyver would create a flap hat; he was a big fan of the show. My mom, ever the anti-fashionista, wore a T-shirt with an image of a duck dressed as Rhett Butler that read, "Frankly my duck, I don't give a quack" (her favorite shirt; she wore it all the time). I could feel better about my appearance compared to them, at least. That is, until my father forced me to wear a Lets Putt tee shirt over my ensemble. Throughout my childhood, I frequently fulfilled the function of a walking billboard, never by choice.

The rounds started, and besides feeling a little toasty under all my layers, I played pretty well. I started eliminating the competition, making my way towards the semi-finals. Unbeknownst to me, television crews had arrived, unannounced, and to my father's obvious giddiness, to film our little tournament for a community story (aka, fluff piece) for the eleven o'clock news. I must have played two whole rounds unaware of their presence. I was so engrossed in winning. But at some point, I looked up to acknowledge the world around me and I spotted the TV camera. I'm sure my mouth dropped low enough to graze the green. I unleashed my inner Wonder Woman quick change powers. If I could have spun around really fast until my clothes changed like Linda Carter's, I would've been a happy girl. I raced inside the clubhouse, to the back office, and found a spare set of shorts and a different color Lets Putt tee. We had tons of the cotton candy-colored shirts lying around; and if there were none in my size, I had to wear them larger; belt them for a flirty, but awful, knit dress. I tore off the ludicrous hat and tossed my hair up into a messy but acceptable pony tail and returned outside to my spot on the course as if nothing had happened. I morphed into a new person. Vanity beat out fear of the sun at this point. This was television we were talking about, people! Local television, which was even better, since people I actually knew would be watching. I only hoped that the camera did not have any shots of my previous get-up. I needed to focus on the game and pray that my sunscreen would do the trick by itself with no other protection.

I won my match and found myself in the semi-finals, a showdown with Marco, to compete in the finals. Marvin had been knocked out by someone with an aggressive personality who had unsettled him, due to his overly meek nature, and thrown him off his game. Steve had succumbed to elimination when one the Lets Putt employees, a pretty high school junior, bent over to pick up a piece of trash she had dropped, just as he prepared to putt. He ended up double bogeying the hole. Bob and Tim would compete for the other spot in the finals. Let's go, boys. Or, rather, much older men, who shouldn't find it dignified to compete against an adolescent girl.

I beat Marco, easily. I don't mean to sound conceited. But in between putts, he decided to commence logic/trivia time, and asked me who was buried in Grant's Tomb (duh!). I pretended to get it wrong, and said, "Napoleon?" (with innocent eyes). This totally caught him off guard, resulting in his next shot resembling a hockey slap shot rather than a golf putt. He kept staring at me as if hoping to find any evidence of my lost intelligence. I turned and smiled to the television cameras. Tim also had luck against Bob and took the match. Bob had been resting his bits and pieces on the Putter Cup, and it must have somehow bunched up his underwear because when he went to make his final putt, he executed a weird kick-out with one leg, in an attempt to straighten his undergarments. His jerking action startled his grip and he ended up putting when I don't think he really meant to right at that point. A shame, really. Not a dignified way to go down. Especially with the eye of the local news watching and a journalist nearby with pen to paper.

The title came down to me and Tim. Or, as I liked to call him, "The Professional." Doing a mental "blow off my nails and buff them on my shirt" (or maybe I actually did this for real; hard to remember with all the pressure), I put my ball on the tee mat and started the round. All of the eliminated players followed us around the course as an eager, yet courteous and quiet, gallery. I aced every hole. I'd never played a game before of straight holes-in-one. My previous best score had topped at twenty-one on a par two course - meaning you would end up with thirty-six if you scored par on every hole; for any of you with a slight math deficiency, like me. But today I stayed on schedule for perfection. Only, Tim matched me shot for shot. I always hear that athletes really bring it when the chips are down. And we lived up to that notion. And don't smirk about the "athletes" bit. Something clearly had to give; one of us had to win and one had to lose. I was determined to win. I tried to size up my opponent in the hopes of finding some advantage. Wasn't he hot in all that polyester? Today he wore green and white; green pants, white polo-style shirt with golf clubs embroidered on the pocket; so that he wore official Lets Putt colors. Little sneak! He was so sure he would win that he wanted to prepare for any photo op. Well I would show him.

By the eighteenth hole we had lost our steam; exhausted. We had both scored a perfect game so far. It seemed we'd already conquered the challenge of the course. To each have an absolute perfect game would be near impossible. I went first on the final hole, and missed. I heard a hissed "yes" from Tim. Nice. Real mature. I made my easy second putt and waited, disappointed. Tim stepped up to the tee, hit his ball, after a much pronounced test swing ritual, and, missed as well. Sweet! He dropped his head down dramatically and his comb-over slipped a little. He trudged up the hill of the hole. He took his time to aim. Like gently slicing the first piece of a wedding cake, he eased the putter next to the ball (except he did this six to eight times, maybe in hopes of creating some sort of groove in the carpet next to the ball that might help him). After about five minutes of this procedure, people started to look at their watches, realizing the inanity of watching a mini-golf showdown and praying for no "sudden death." He finally hit the ball to try to make the three and a half foot putt. He missed. He thudded to his knees, head towards the heavens in agony and a look of "why?" I don't think he actually said the word but you could just tell that's what he wanted to say. Then he dropped his head, his hands covering his face. I started jumping up and down. The thirteen-year-old champ. I had trumped him with my score of nineteen.

The local news station later that night showed me smiling, holding my trophy with the lady on top. A nice touch. The local paper ran a picture of Tim down on his knees beside a photo of me grinning with my bouncy pony tail, in a sort of weird thrill-of-victory-and-agony-of-defeat layout. I, of course, looked great, since I represented the thrill of victory side of the equation.

Unfortunately, both news outlets also showed shots from earlier in the night of early favorites in the competition. My flap hat seemed to play an overly significant role in these shots. There was no name attached to the tag line, just "early hopefuls." Hopefully nobody put two and two together. You will be happy to know that I vowed off flap hats for the rest of my existence. I guess I'm too vain to risk that kind of exposure again. However, my fear of skin cancer would continue to stick around. I just make it a habit to get checked annually and keep myself protected in a more normal way. I'm sure the people around me appreciate this decision.

Hypochondriac Lesson #4:
You will not die from every health problem.

Sub-Lesson: Don't ever sit in a fire ant bed.

## 4- *I'm on a High Kick to Hell*

"I made it! I made it! I MADE IT!" I screamed. But only on the inside. On the outside, I sat perfectly upright and silent at my traditional one-piece wooden school desk, totally composed. Dignified, really. I saw her walk in. The Drill Team Officer. The ritual occurred as follows: about a hundred of us broke our bodies and bruised our skin trying out for a week, then the sadists made us wait another week, biting our nails down to bare rawness, critically analyzing every possible mistake we could've made. On a vomit-inducing Friday morning, they quietly entered your first period class if you were one of the select twenty-five who made the team, and pinned a little white cowboy boot to your shirt; part of the signature costume of teeny tiny red pleated skirt, white dress shirt, red fitted vest, black bowtie, black top hat and white boots. Smokin' hot. It was the dream. The Longwood Senior High School Drill Team, comprised of seventy-five precision high-kickers; just like my beloved Rockettes. I wanted this so badly, I could practically smell the ink of my name written in sharpie on the little paper boot badge. The Officer smiled right at me, a welcome sight after the torture of try-outs, and I could taste victory like my salty sweat. I sat up straighter (Drill Team members had perfect posture) and she walked right by me to Heather Shafer, who immediately burst into tears, amid a round of tepid class applause. It was early morning; the rest of the students could barely keep their eyes open. I slumped down, defeated, and probably frowning rather obviously; no sour grapes for Heather Shafer or anything.

"Kat, I'm so sorry you didn't make it," Heather said, whisper-crying, as the Geometry teacher sidled up to her desk with a box of tissues. Tissues of joy for Heather. She held the box out to me and raised her eyebrows in question. Tears of sorrow for you, Kat? I waved her away with a weak smile. I would not cry in front

of my whole class, whether happy or sad. I just looked around and shrugged, as if

to say, "Hey, it doesn't matter. Comme çi, comme ça. No big deal. Didn't really

want it anyway." I put my elbow on my desk and rested my heavy head, and heart,

in my hand. The teacher went back to her lecture, although her voice began to

fade into unintelligible sounds like the teacher on Charlie Brown. I couldn't focus

on math. Only the ticking clock, which showed I had just five minutes left of class

and therefore five minutes left of a chance. But they'd come around so early for

Heather, so really, no chance. Sad!

But wait. What's this? I heard the sound of running feet down the hall

outside the door. Two Officers came busting through at the same time, acting

out of breath, but not really; they were so in shape. Interrupting class again, they

walked through the room, but this time, straight to me. My spirits soared like my

highest kick to date - pretty high, I'm still sore; in fact, I think I might've pulled

something. They pinned the little boot on me and pulled me up into a group

embrace. We were sisters of the Drill Team, now. My new friends. Heather cried

again. My teacher came back around with the tissues. I took one and dabbed my

eyes, even though they were dry. I'm not a big crier. But I didn't want anyone to

think I lacked emotion or appreciation. Heather jumped up and joined the girl

hug, until my teacher finally tapped on the chalk board in a call to order. Enough.

She had homework to give. The Officers bounced out of the room. I couldn't stop

grinning. What a glorious day. High school would now turn totally awesome.


\*\*\*\*

"What...are you STUPID or something? Do you even have a brain in your

HEAD?" I could feel her angry, hot breath on my face. Thank heavens she'd recently ingested something minty fresh.

"I do have a...." (I wanted to say, "I do have a brain because it's melting in this bleeping HEAT!)

"What? Are you talking back to me?" I stared at her. She clearly did not want an answer so I waited. "You don't talk to me. You just do what I SAY! And that seems to be beyond your capabilities." I disgusted her. "You disgust me!" See. I'd heard it before, so I knew her next words as if I had telepathy. She was the Co-Captain and I was, well, according to her I was, "DISGUSTING. I don't even know how you made this TEAM!" Pleasant.

I tried to remain calm, look her in the eye, but my stomach hurt so badly. I couldn't tell if I had just overworked my muscles or if I had eaten the wrong thing at lunch. Who am I kidding? I hadn't eaten anything at all that day; so rattled with nerves. I darted my eyes around. I could see all the other newbies like me, on the wrong side of a verbal whipping, all uniformly standing at attention with their arms behind their backs. We were dancing our way through drill team camp, held at a local university; a supposed bonding trip for the new team. Learn some moves, make some friends, perform at the end for an audience of proud parents. Yeah right! Our group decided to remove itself from the other teams, practicing out behind a building in a remote parking lot, so that our officers could berate us without fear of repercussions. We were the best team; we had the annual plaques to prove it. But our faces held the haunted expressions of abused puppies.

I really wished Co-Captain would get out of my face. Her menacing fire made standing in the July sun feel like a living cremation. The pain in my stomach rose, lava-like into my esophagus.

"You better pay attention to me," she said, seething, a small speckle of spittle landing on my chin. "I swear to you that you won't perform once this season if you don't shape up."

I tried to nod that I understood, even attempted a smile, but instead doubled over violently, throwing up all over her feet. Ahh. So that explained the stomach pain. Is it bad that it gave me some tiny bit of pleasure to watch her leap backwards, arms flying reflexively, as if electrocuted? I retched again; so much better, yet somehow worse. My heart felt like a baby bird trying for the first time to fly, beating fast yet weak at the same time. Co-Captain grabbed my arm and raced me away from the rest of the team; in case my bad sportsmanship or laziness was contagious. The teamed viewed illness as a deterrent to dancing and completely the dancer's fault. She ushered me into a bathroom in an empty classroom building and started trying to clean me up. The public bathroom smell, bleach and chlorine, like a bathroom at a water park, caused my abdomen to clench yet again. I caught a glimpse of myself in the mirror. Ashen. Stony. Gray. Not a healthy look for a teenage girl, much less a glamorous precision dancer in training. She splashed water on my face in bucket scoops created by her hands. I got the impression she enjoyed throwing something at me, even if it served to make me feel better. Then she pulled four or five paper towels from the dispenser in quick succession and dabbed at my face and neck, almost maternally. Maybe she had a heart after all.

"Are you okay?" she asked, in dare I say, a rather concerned way.

"Um, I don't know. I think so." I felt dizzy, actually. "I think I need to sit down." She pursed her lips, the concern starting to evaporate like my sweat in the air conditioning. Soon all traces would disappear. As if all in my imagination.

"You have five minutes. FIVE!" She held up her hand with all fingers spread out, in case I couldn't remember how to determine five. "Then I expect you back out in that line with the rest of the idiots." She executed a precise about-face and sternly exited the bathroom, leaving me to regain my composure and hopefully a normal heart rate. I splashed more cold water in my face. Turning the faucet as cold as it would go, I leaned over and drank straight from the stream of water. I could've stayed that way for days. Who knew that drill team camp could simulate desert travel? I felt like I could drink for eternity, especially to wash away the horrible stomach acid that saturated my taste buds. What I wouldn't give for a rain storm to blow in and force us to go inside, or at least cool the world down for a minute. Nothing says fun like dancing on asphalt with the temperature around a hundred degrees. I guess Co-Captain eagerly awaited my return to the festivities, and I must've taken longer than five minutes, because the bathroom door flung open and she blew in, ablaze.

"You're DONE. Let's go." She pointed at the door and I weakly stumbled through. Nobody feels strong when dehydrated; especially after vomiting repeatedly. Co-Captain apparently didn't get that memo. "Did you just think you could get out of it that easily? '*Oh look, I threw up. I'm so sick.*' Well nice try, but no such luck. You WILL perform and you WILL get the blue ribbon. Anything else and you're out for the season. Got it?" Yes indeed. All clear. And the amazing thing? I did manage to pull it off. I couldn't eat and I had to go to bed early, missing good gossip time (probably mostly about me anyway, so I guess it didn't matter), but I gathered myself up the next day and performed. My head spun, sure, and a sharp pain radiated around my midsection. My heart rate still had not slowed to normal, but I was trying to perform after all. I couldn't help but notice that these symptoms hadn't visited any of my teammates. What was wrong with me? I'd been dancing for years. Why was I the only one getting sick? I didn't enjoy the doubts that nested in my brain like a colony of hornets. I tried to shove those fears to the back of my mind and just smiled the whole time, pretending to have a blast. At the end of the routine, we put our hands behind our backs, closed our eyes and waited for ribbon distribution. As noted before, the Officers simply prohibited us from earning anything but blue. Even though I had nothing left in my body to heave, I felt that I might anyway while I waited for the judge's hand to place the ribbon in my own. I sucked in breath when I felt the satin on my palm.

"Okay, ladies. Take a look at your ribbons," said the announcer. I slowly brought my hand around and opened one eye at a time. Blue. Thank the high heavens. I heard an agonizing shriek as another new member discovered a red ribbon in her hand. My last thought was a selfish, "Thank God that's not me." I collapsed onto the floor. That couldn't be a good sign. My body just gave up. My parents hurried down the bleachers of the gym and picked me up by my arms.

"Are you alright?" My mother looked worried. My father looked strangely pleased.

"I'm fine. I think I'm fine." I used them as support to hold myself up, feeling ridiculous. I didn't have a broken leg, yet that's how they hauled me out of the gym. The Drill Team Officers would surely have a field day talking about me later. Paranoid? Of course. But let's be serious. We're talking about teenage girls here. And I was the ONLY one who had a problem. Although Red Ribbon Girl would surely come in a close second in their feeding frenzy.

My mom pulled a bottle out of her bag. Gatorade. Oh sweet nectar! Once they got my invalid self into the car, I guzzled the orange elixir, feeling my electrolytes replenish, imagining my sickly, shriveled cells plumpen on the spot. I felt better already. My father had started talking but I barely registered his words.

"….great news. Are you ready?"

"mmm, hmmm," I said, absentmindedly.

"We're pregnant! You're going to have a little brother or sister." *What!?*

"Yeah, I'd been so sick. I thought I might have stomach cancer," said my mother. See, looking back, it's painfully clear that my little problem with health fears just might've run in the family. "But when I went to the doctor, he said 'I have good news, and I have interesting news. The good news is you don't have stomach cancer. The interesting news is that you're pregnant.' At thirty-eight! Can you believe that?"

No, I couldn't believe that. Back then, and where I lived, people my parents' age did not have babies. Funny how thirty-eight is so common now for even first-time moms; but certainly not in my neighborhood growing up. My first thought? "My parents have sex?" Ugh. Next thought. High school wasn't getting as awesome as I had first expected. It was just getting weird.

\*\*\*

"Welcome to Band Camp," the band leader yelled into the megaphone to scattered applause. Some over-enthusiastic "woo hoo"s, and a general buzz of excitement among most of the young crowd permeated the humid August atmosphere.

We sat by groups on the football field. There was the Marching Band; the hundred or so musicians in the school willing to wear pleated maroon polyester pants and strange shaped hats in public once a week; the Flag Corps; usually the overweight girls who couldn't make either the Cheerleading Squad or the Drill Team; the Baton Twirlers; obvious misfits living in their own little sequined leotard clique of two; and us, the Drill Team; sitting in rigid formation slightly further away than necessary from the group, in a subliminal hope of avoiding too much interaction with those viewed as inferior. There might've been an actual fear that "band geekiness" was contagious. I'm not saying this was me. I had plenty of band friends; just pointing out the group pathology. None of the clapping or happy exclamations came from our group. Band camp proved a necessary evil, tolerated grudgingly, that led to halftime performance glory, when our kick line would take the spotlight at the front. All eyes would then fall on us. During this week, however, we had to mingle with the masses and pretend we operated as performance equals. This elitist attitude came with the package as soon as the boot badge first took its spot on our shirts. And since, strangely, no one ever contradicted our superior claims, we could run with it. A pretty swell idea for teenage girls.

After the debacle of Drill Team camp the previous month, I didn't relish another week on a hot field. I had heard the horror stories from previous years, mostly from outsiders like those band friends I mentioned, who witnessed the treachery first hand. Of course Drill Team members never spoke ill of other Drill Team member practices, even if said practices were violent or could easily qualify as assault and/or battery. We all had a healthy fear of repeat abuse and repercussions. The theory was, if you stayed quiet, you might squeak by under the radar. But outside witnesses seemed to have an endless supply of tales of hazing and other physical trials. I thought they probably exaggerated just because we didn't have hourly group hand stacking and high fives like them, who seemed so happy, and relaxed. Were they actually having fun? Imagine having so much fun in a high school activity. What a waste! (The world, according to Drill Team).

While the other groups galloped and galavanted onto the field in the morning and after breaks, we emerged from our organized spot on the bleachers in a single file line, hands behind our backs, as usual, with our large water cooler jugs banging painfully against our tail bones. In perfect formation, we seamlessly deposited our water jugs by the track fence and continued to our spots on the field, never breaking stride or character. Our Drill Team persona never waivered. Most, although not all, of us were fairly pleasant people under different circumstances. We kept the rigidity up as part of the character. The other groups watched our serpentine line approach with dazzled amazement; and sympathy. The practices began and that's when I descended into my personal summer vacation in Hell.

Co-Captain moved right in my face, again, as if magnetized. I give her high marks for bravery, considering the voluminous splashing she received from my insides during our last encounter, like sitting in the front row at a dolphin show, if Flipper had eaten a few bad fish.

"Today, I'm not goin' to take your crap," she whispered in my ear. Well, okay. Wrong end, but who's really keeping track?

I nodded almost imperceptibly. She eyed me with warning. That's right. I better understand.

I went along with the motions, making sure I landed where designated as the band played the theme song from Robin Hood: Prince of Thieves. At least, I think that's what they tried to play. It sounded more like a warble at times. But I couldn't fault them. It was burning hot. And the instruments probably suffered as well.

Each time I messed up, I received punishment.

"Just for that, you get no water at the next break." Good thinking. At this point, you might wonder, "Where's the coach, the adult in all this?" Good question. She, herself, was ex-military of some sort and had little tolerance for weakness. She believed in tough love, just without the actual love part. She put full faith in her handpicked Officers and basically turned her back so that she wouldn't see what they inflicted on the members. Therefore, in her mind, if not a court of law, she would not be culpable. I'm glad the high school paid her to do this.

I noticed I wasn't the only one receiving admonishment. I watched as a new member named Bridgitte turned slightly left before realizing that she needed to go to the right. While she quickly corrected herself, Captain jumped on top of her in an instant, ready to debase. Captain, a blond bombshell who looked eerily similar to the Princess Bride (which sadly still makes that movie difficult for me to watch to this day), brought over a sunscreen stick; the kind that you painted brightly on your face like surf war paint; and wrote "Moron" across her forehead. Bridgitte took it like a champ, having no idea that the writing would remain on her head for a week after the humiliation, in sunburned exposure, forcing her to cry and wear a hat, so her parents wouldn't see, until her skin peeled and faded.

Next, Heather Shafer subjected herself to a lashing. She actually turned around a couple of beats too soon and ended up staring an Officer right in the face. Unable to hide the mistake in any way, Heather braced herself for the worst. Officer brought over tin foil. Since I could ascertain no other purpose for the foil; we weren't cooking or storing anything; I deduced that the sole reason was to degrade. Heather stood at attention as Officer formulated a creative hat of silver on her head, antennae sticking out like a deformed alien as imagined by a small child in the fifties, just right for allowing the sun to broil poor Heather to perfection. Well done. It amazes me that Heather made it through the day under such duress. What strength. I'll always admire her for that.

I didn't fare quite as well. After about two hours on the field and repeated denials of water, I started to feel a little like road kill. Run over, trampled and flattened. I was only missing the bloody guts, but felt it was just a matter of time. Co-Captain seemed to smell my defeat, or maybe it was more the rising bile. Before I knew it she imposed herself into my personal space again. I listened and then I didn't. I found myself occupied with the strange gray haze growing around

Co-Captain's head. I could still hear her words, but vaguely. They sounded as if projected through a long tunnel or a poor overseas phone connection. I remember squinting to try to see her better. Strange since I'm sure, given our history, that she only stood mere inches away.

"…wrong with you?"

Knees locked, still at attention, I went completely deaf, then completely blind. I woke up under a tent off to the side of the field, cold rag on my forehead and Heather Shafer sitting quietly towards a corner near the pole. Guess she didn't want to catch what I had.

"What happened?" I asked, feeling like I wasn't ready to wake or even sit up. "How did I get over here?" My heart raced and my tongue stuck to the roof of my mouth like fly paper.

"You fainted. I can't believe you did that! You are so not going to perform this season," she said, more incredulous at my apparent insubordination than concerned for my well-being. "Captain and Co-Captain had to carry you over here themselves. You are in SO much trouble." I couldn't help but smile a little at the thought of that sight. I'm surprised they didn't drop me a couple of times just for the fun of it. But Heather seemed very serious about this issue.

"I didn't do it on purpose. Aach!" I grabbed at my head as I sat up. It felt like a bowling ball had made a strike right on it. I composed myself into a seated position but had my knees bent up to my chest. My stomach hurt severely and this position did nothing to soothe. I really didn't want to throw up again. I had started developing a reputation, and not the cool one that all teenagers desire. Barfing and passing out from overheating does not lead to a place on the Homecoming Court.

"Well, maybe not, but you should try to control yourself better."

"Again, I didn't do it on purpose. I can't CONTROL it! Do you think I enjoy this?" She looked out towards the field, pensively. She DID think I enjoyed this.

"All I know is that you get to sit on the side a lot while the rest of us have to be out there the whole time." She pointed aggressively toward the field. Maybe she was just sorry she hadn't thought of fainting or puking, herself. "It's not fair." Harsh. She thought I'd made it all up. But wait.

"Wait. What are you doing here, then? It seems to me that you're also sitting out at the moment." Ha!

"Because of this stupid tin foil on my head, I think they thought I might faint, too. Like you. So they told me to take a few minutes and make sure you woke up." How thoughtful of them. And if I didn't wake up? Were there alternative arrangements for that? Or did they just want the information either way for logistics purposes? I looked at Heather and felt bad for her. I hoped that she wouldn't faint and feel this way. I was scared. I didn't feel right. My heart wouldn't slow down and I had a sick stomach and general wooziness.

"Oh, and they made me call your parents. Your mom's on her way." She smacked her lips, annoyed. "You're so lucky. You probably get to go home." Things are pretty bad when the other girls consider you lucky for passing out or throwing up, instead of staying on the field for an extracurricular activity. "Since you're fine, I'm going back out there." I would debate the definition of "fine" but I waved at her anyway.

"Good luck." She trotted off with her hands behind her back, silver antennae bouncing ludicrously with each step.

I felt like death but I have to admit, I enjoyed sitting under this shade even if the heat continued its oppressive quest to control us all. Over a hundred degrees at this point. But at least the sun had stopped beating down directly on my head. I started to experience a prickly sensation on the back of my thighs; my rear-end actually; and at first thought that maybe I had incurred circulation issues from fainting then trying to get up too fast. I remembered my mom's little talk about my black out when I got up too fast from falling at my dance recital all those years ago. But no, this started to feel less like minor pins and needles and more like, well, major pins and needles. Stinging, painful, then grotesquely itching pins and needles.

I looked down slowly as I couldn't move very fast at this point, and almost fainted again. I tried to scramble to my feet, then fell again right in the same spot. The worst spot humanly possible for bare skin to rest. A small dirt mound inhabited by one of Florida's many invasive insect inhabitants- the red fire ant. I was sweaty and slippery and couldn't get my footing and kept falling right back into my horrible nightmare. I could feel them all over the backs of my thighs and crawling around in my shorts; little stripey nylon short shorts, a la Richard Simmons. Oh my God. They were creeping into my nether regions. How do you treat them up and around there? I finally mustered the strength, like those people who can lift cars to save people's lives, and started spinning frantically around like a dog chasing its tail, trying to brush the satanic creatures off my body. The stinging brought tears to my eyes; or, at least it would've if I wasn't dehydrated. I cried dryly, trying to clear myself of this affliction. The group on the field noticed something awry and looked over just in time to see me with my hands down my pants, swishing them rapidly around in a kind of spastic dance. They might have thought I was mocking them (*Hey look at me. I'm just pretending to be sick so I can sit in the shade*) because it took them a long while to send someone over to determine my problem. I knew that I screamed but my voice came out in a hoarse garble. Maybe they understood when they saw me grab my water jug, pull the elastic waist of my shorts out about a foot and douse myself with fluid. Yeah, that can't be right, better see if she's gone mental.

Co-Captain walked with purpose towards me. Surely she would understand that I had a serious problem. Let's face it, she and Captain laid me on or near that terrible colony to begin with. Just as she neared the shade tent, my mother ran through the gates and to my rescue.

Co-Captain stopped and just waved at my mother. As my mother helped me out towards the car, I swear I could hear Co-Captain say, "Good riddance."


"Okay, I'm going to draw some blood and see what we're looking at," said the Doctor. "And I'll get the nurse in here to put some ointment on those bites. You must have about fifty of them." I nodded at him, lacking the energy to even speak. Terror enveloped me. I know I had read somewhere about a person who received so many bug bites that they couldn't survive the build-up of poison that coursed through their veins from the creatures and had died. If only I could remember the culprit bug. Please don't let it be fire ants. And please, just bring me some relief. I looked like a helpless nine-year-old sitting on the examining table with my legs dangling over the side; pale and drawn. I had seen my reflection in a paper towel dispenser in the room and I looked sick.

The nurse came in with all of her equipment and went to work to draw my blood. I wasn't sure what they were looking for, but it can never be good, right? My mom tried to lighten the mood by talking about going back-to-school clothes shopping, but it didn't help. A nurse tied a rubber band around my arm. Even new fashion couldn't cheer me up or distract me from the next steps. I felt the cold of the alcohol as the nurse swabbed my arm to make it sterile.

"Here we go," she said. I stared straight ahead, right at a "hang loose"-cute-cat-hanging-from-a-tree-limb poster. She injected the needle into what I refer to as my elbow pit. The last words I heard were, "Wait. Don't hold your breath!"

I woke sometime later looking up to multiple unfamiliar faces; two holding my legs, one waving smelling salts under my nose. I started gagging. That stuff punctures your nasal cavity with its Zeus-like strength.

"Wow, look how the color just came right back to her face," said one nurse, and they all laughed. I looked over at my mother and she had her head down, shaking it from side to side in obvious embarrassment.

"Mom, do you love me?" She wouldn't answer me. Just kept shaking her head. Does that mean "No?" I'd done it now. My own mother couldn't even bring herself to look at me. I did notice that my legs and backside felt a little better and once I could raise myself up on the table a small degree I could see that my legs had a sheen, like the nurses had covered them in Crisco. I have come to realize that ointments are wonderful things. Relief in a tube. The doctor came back in to discuss my prognosis.

"Kat, let's start with the ant bites. It's my recommendation that you stay off of ant hills." He smiled, clearly pleased with himself and his vast humor. You can't learn that apparent, uh, skill, in medical school. Considering I had just fainted for the second time in one day (maybe I did have the vapors), I felt in no mood for his jokes. When I continued to glare at him, he cleared his throat and moved on. "But the bites will be fine. They'll be uncomfortable for a while but just keep putting this cream on them and it'll help." He sighed and ran his hand through his hair. Was that sanitary?

"As for your spell today, it's pretty clearly the result of heat exhaustion. Some people tolerate the heat better than others. Your recent history suggests that you're not one of those people." He went to medical school for that? "But heat exhaustion can be very serious. You put yourself repeatedly through what you did today and you'll wind up in the hospital with heat stroke." As if that weren't enough to put a damper on my day, he iced the cake with this little gem, "No more band camp for you."

"But wait! I can't be on the team if I don't go to band camp. How will I learn what to do on the field?" My mother patted my arm, to comfort and tell me to shut up. The doctor thought silently for what seemed like twenty minutes.

"Okay, look. If you insist on going back out there, I'll write you a note and you can go. But only to observe. Under no circumstances are you to get back out on that field. Understood?" I guess that's the best we could do.

I spent the rest of the week on the sidelines, under the shade tent, in shame, Doctor's note in hand. It did little to sway the group that I had a real problem. They still thought I had finagled my way into a free pass. But I worried about something more. Heat Stroke. Stroke. I was only a young girl. Those sorts of things weren't supposed to affect me. I was supposed to be invincible, like a superhero. Strong. I was more scared than a mouse in a lion's cage.

I would like to say that I would get better with the heat over time, but the truth is that I still have a hard time spending prolonged periods in the direct sun on a hot summer day. I think the heat traps itself in my thick dark hair and I start to feel my head sizzling, much like I imagined Heather's cooking under the tin foil that day. Her prediction about my performance schedule pretty much came true. I didn't get to perform as much as I would've liked. In fact, the only time I got to don those sweet white cowboy boots was when they deemed another member too fat to perform, after mandatory weekly weigh-ins, and I then measured marginally less disgusting than her. It was exhilarating. But after I hung up my top hat from my big debut, I decided to place my talents and energies into other high school activities. Besides, I figured my mother shouldn't have to spend so much time worrying about me or physically picking me up off the ground in her newly

pregnant state.

Hypochondriac Lesson #5:
Don't let your mind make your body go nuts.

*5- Oral Fixation*

I was sweet fifteen and never been kissed. I know, I know. The saying says "sweet sixteen." But where I grew up, no kissing by fifteen meant you could head straight to spinsterhood. Grab a few cats along the way. Put on your bathrobe and be sure to take that tub of ice cream. Does that mean that the girls at my high school let go of their virtue easily? I guess at any high school some girls will give it up without a fight, while others will hang on to their chastity until they meet "the one." I didn't really fall into either one of these categories. I had no moral objection to physical affection of any kind. Well, I'm sure there are plenty of things I might've found objectionable, but in my innocence, I wouldn't have thought of those things. Geez, get your mind out of the gutter. Basically, I just hadn't encountered the right opportunity. A classic case of harboring interest in the males who wouldn't give me a second look, and brushing aside the boys who expressed interest in me. Therefore, there I was; sweet fifteen and never been kissed. But hopeful.

A couple of components in my life worked in my favor to provide opportunity for me to reach the destination of a coveted lip lock. For one, previous membership on the Drill Team guaranteed that at least a few boys would ask for my phone number. But I cared very little about these obvious pursuers. I mean, please, I get no glances from them for the past eight years (we all went to elementary and middle school together), but Kat makes the Drill Team, wears sexy tights around school, and suddenly has the attention of multiple suitors. Suspect, to say the least. I wanted a relationship with at least some sort of true basis to it other than my social status; as true as kids can achieve in the young years of hormonal upheaval and loyalties that ebb and flow, like storm surges.

My family's ownership of Lets Putt America made up the other fortunate circumstance. As I noted before, my father only hired the hottest, most lusted-after individuals from the high school, both male and female. This gave me a unique position to mingle with the cute boys I otherwise wouldn't have known. There might've even been times that I would purposely ASK my dad to put me on the schedule if it meant I could work side-by-side with a locally regarded heartthrob. I might've even; hypothetically, I can neither confirm nor deny; swayed my father's decisions to hire certain individuals. Either way, I had the special opportunity to spend a great deal of quality time with some serious studs. My prospects improved.

Of course, I then abandoned the Drill Team to pursue more cerebral, and indoor, activities. I joined the Debate Team. This didn't convey upon me the same social status or provide quite the draw that skimpy clothing held. But I secretly loved smart guys. This wasn't the usual thing you admit at teenage slumber parties. Abs always trump IQ in youthful group settings. But I enjoyed debate and pursued it with much flourish. I generally lived by the notion that I would eventually turn into a star lawyer. My father and I worshiped Perry Mason, waiting eagerly for each TV-length movie, and I was the youngest person I knew, by at least three decades, with a Matlock obsession. Plus, I could seriously formulate an argument. My parents were annoyed with me, I'm sure, when I would stump them with my logic. Or perhaps I had just beaten them down enough with my incessant talking, and in fatigue, they would relent. No way to tell for sure. Debate gave me an outlet to always feel right. I loved every minute of it.

So where did this leave me with my kissing quest; my osculatory endeavor? Better than once imagined, yet having an unanticipated reaction. Here's how it went down. The previous summer I'd voluntarily participated in a physical education class in summer school, in order to avoid entirely any discomfort during the school year of dressing out in horrible P.E. uniforms, running up and down the stadium stairs, then heading to my next class either a sweaty mess if I didn't shower, or a wet mess with hair issues if I did shower. I felt that summer school presented the best option to meet the mandatory PE requirement with minimal effort. Three weeks and done. Shazam! And I should note that the school board applied the term, "physical education," very loosely to the curriculum of this course. Mondays and Wednesdays we went to the bowling alley. Now I don't know about you, but it's a rare occurrence, unless sick and feverish, that you break a sweat while bowling. Tuesdays and Thursdays we spent half the day in the weight room, the girls sitting in clusters on the floor watching the football players training for the fall and other males working out on the weight machines. The girls produced lots of "ohmigod, he's so hot" types of conversations. The second half of those days we ventured into the gym to watch the athletes play shirts vs. skins indoor games. Our male classmates joined the girl clusters on the sidelines at that point as they were generally not invited to join the ball players. More ogling ensued.

I usually had no interest in the beefcake, weight lifting, "I'm so cut," type of guy. But as with most things, exceptions exist to every rule. One football player stuck out to me, pulling me in like gravity. When I watched the scrimmages, the other players looked blurred while I saw him perfectly clearly. I won't say he had a light around him that might have emanated from within like an angel because that would sound cheesy (ahem), but I will say, very frankly, I found him attractive and thought I might like to get to know him. As a person. Aside from his obvious physical attributes. It's all about what's on the inside, right? And I knew that if given the chance, we would get along famously, like macaroni and cheese, chips and salsa, prosciutto and melon (more upscale but still a delicious duo).

What started as boring summer school, soon developed into, "I can't wait until Tuesday and Thursday" school. I relished each shirts vs. skins event, especially when He drew the straw for skins. At this point, I didn't even know his name. I watched as if immersed in the Super Bowl, cheering with fervor, laughing with my friends so that if He looked over He would think, "Wow, she must have a great sense of humor; look at her laughing." Or maybe, "Wow, she has a lot of friends, she must be fun to hang out with." That kind of thing. I was working it, in really no way at all. Then one day something unbelievable and quite memorable happened. He ran to catch the ball thrown in his direction, stumbled out of the boundary line, and because of sweaty floors, slid over towards me, lost his balance and fell right on top of me. The spikiness of his dirty blond hair slammed right into my chin, causing me to bite my tongue. Even though I could taste blood, I barely noticed because his face landed so close to mine; so close I could see his pores. Oh mercy. I'm not a huge lover of sweat, in fact I usually find it quite abhorrent, but his sweat smelled good. Almost magical; like honey and sunshine and man. The fact that he'd essentially knocked the breath out of me fazed me not in the slightest. I could've stayed that way for the rest of class, no problem. Then he did something else remarkable. He looked me right in the eye as he got up and said, "Sorry. Are you okay?" I felt my heart skip a beat. Then four or ten. That didn't feel quite right. Strange, but He more than took my mind off the uneasy, foreign feeling. This must be what all the songs talk about. "*You make my heart go giddyup.*" I think I might've said something riveting like, "Mmm hmm." But he was gone, back to the game before he likely heard this stunning response. It doesn't change the fact that this Adonis spoke to me. ME! Well, this summer school class was definitely worth the effort of waking up in the morning. My only regret? That I never learned his name before the three week class ended.

That happened during the summer. Now I was invested in the school year and in preparations for my first debate tournament just two weeks away. I had gotten to know the rest of the team pretty well and I couldn't wait to go on an extended overnight field trip, so that we could have a cool bonding experience and be able to share inside jokes in the hallway. I might've been over-thinking this just a bit. Each day after school, my mom picked me up and took me to Lets Putt, where I would do my homework, and in this case, prepare my opening arguments without too much interruption while my parents worked the business.

I remember one specific day well above the others in this monotonous routine. I sat at a small round table, the standard size of tables in an ice cream parlor, with curly-cue metal frame chairs to match. I could hear the clicking of the adding machine from the office, as my mom handled all the books and numbers. Luckily it was just clicking and not horrible retching coming from my mother, as her morning sickness issues had finally subsided once she reached her second trimester of pregnancy. My dad stood at the counter, quietly filling in the schedule, a more laborious than expected task each week, given the high demand of popular teenagers' time. From him I could only hear the scratches of pencil on the paper against a Formica countertop, followed by irritated eraser rubbing when a scheduling decision wouldn't work out. I can't tell you how many times the cheerleaders would simply not work with a football player after a bad break-up. The sound of crunching M&M's from the frozen yogurt topping bar emanated from my father at fairly regular intervals. I could vaguely hear the PA system outside, playing oldies but goodies to an empty golf course, as if hoping that the music alone would attract people to the fun. I tried to tune out these noises to focus exclusively on my index cards, practicing saying my argument in a whisper while trying to avoid looking directly at the cards. I was talking to myself. And that's when He walked in.

So engrossed in my own activity, I barely noticed the noise of the squeaky hinges as the front door opened to our clubhouse. My dad refused to fix the squeak, because at least he would always know when a customer had arrived. Why pay money for a little bell when a faulty door does the trick by itself? I felt a breeze as the person walked in front of my table up to the counter. Still, I didn't pay much attention as my father boomed his greeting, "HI, WELCOME TO LETS PUTT AMERICA. WHAT CAN I DO FOR YOU TODAY? GOLF, GO CARTS, OR YOGURT?" Always, to everyone, and never at a lower volume. I'm not lying when I say that he startled at least three or four people a day, conservatively.

"Hi, yes, I wanted to see if you were hiring." Wait a minute. I recognized that voice. It took me a second to put two and two together, but then my head involuntarily shot up. I felt my face flush as I looked at the back of him.

"What's your name, son?" asked my dad. He would never commit to either "Yes, we're hiring" or "No, sorry, not right now". He was always, or never hiring, depending on whether he liked what he saw.

"Nick. Nick Smith." He suddenly sounded nervous.

"Well, Nick. I assume you're in high school, right?"

"Yes, sir." Nice. Polite. I knew he'd already scored points. It's amazing how many teenagers have no idea about common courtesy, even during a job interview.

"What do you do over there, Nick?"

"Well, I'm a senior and I play football."

"I see. I see. So this means you can't work on Friday nights, then, huh?" He seemed displeased, but I knew he was grinning on the inside as he reached over the cash register to grab an application for Nick. So yes, we were hiring, it seems.

I felt all sorts of clichéd but nevertheless accurately described little butterflies fluttering around my stomach. "Do you know my daughter, Kat?" My dad pointed over at the table to me, and Nick turned, before I had a chance to compose myself and my premature elation at his working status. Nick furrowed his brow as I smiled stupidly. I might've had part of my tongue out. I might also have been doing a silent "Yes" with my elbow into my side, hand made into a fist. All in all not a good look when he peered over at me. Did he furrow because he had no knowledge of me, or because he was trying to decide if I belonged in a special education class and didn't know how to properly react?

"No, I don't think we've met. Do you go to my high school?" Clearly his fall on me had been more memorable to me than to him. But hey, that's okay. I knew his name now.

"Mmm hmm." Why bother changing up the conversation? I would just stick with what I'd said to him in the past. Perhaps my stimulating conversational skill would jar his memory. He nodded, then seeing he wouldn't get anything more from me other than my frozen, and now probably very bizarre, grin, wrinkled his brow and turned back to my dad.

"Fill this out, Nick. Bring it back in the next couple of days, and we'll see if we have anything open in the schedule."

"Really? Thanks, sir." My father beamed at his polite language, and Nick directed a small, and possibly obligatory, little wave in my direction as he walked out.

"Well, what do you think?" My father stared at me, smug twist to his lips. I still gazed out the door wistfully. But this was serious. I needed to get control over myself.

"Dad, I think he would make an excellent addition to the team."

"Really? You don't think we've had too many football players? I'm thinking we need to get some chorus people, or just somebody else to mix it up a bit." He'd better be pulling my leg.

"You have to hire him!" Well, that didn't come out as gracefully as I'd planned. So much for control.

"Oh settle down. Of course I'll hire him. He's a hunk." Yes, my father actually said that. "And stop being so obvious. You'll make a fool out of yourself."

Days later, Nick Smith officially went on the family payroll and into my web of seduction. That was the idea anyway.

**\*\*\***

My father, that little peach, scheduled me with Nick for almost all of the same shifts. I'll always love him for that, no matter what differences we had in life. Working in a fun, youth-centric, environment can bring even the most different people together. It can also serve as the only way two people ever meet, even though they travel the same hallways every single day. Given this wonderful chance, it turned out that Nick and I clicked really well. He was fun and hilarious, and not in an, "I am over-laughing at every unfunny thing he says because I think he's cute" kind of way. Nick had genuine wit. And I genuinely started to like him. A lot. My father grew concerned. He'd never seen me in such a state. He began to tinker with the schedule a little.

"I don't want any more grab assin' at work," he said. While I'm sure that my father did not coin the term, "grab assin'," he deserved recognition for keeping it in play with such frequency. "I'm paying Nick to work, not flirt with my daughter."

"He's not flirting with me," I said, with an obvious smile. So, the flirting was not all in my head. A third party acknowledgment of flirting made it the real deal.

"Yes, he is. And you know it. And you also know that he has a girlfriend."

(Insert car brake squeals and skidding sounds that you might hear in a movie). Oh, what? I didn't tell you he had a girlfriend? Right. The one major roadblock to the whole affair. The Club on the steering wheel of love. The girlfriend. Her name was Chris. Not Christina, or Christy. Just an androgynous Chris. Her father owned one of the most profitable car dealerships in the area and she was loaded. She also kept a ferret as a pet, and would sometimes stop by, much to my chagrin, with the weasely thing on a leash. Nick had been with her for about eight months and complained non-stop about her to me.

"So why don't you break up with her, then," I said, helpfully, on those occasions.

"I don't know. We've been together for a while and she's spent a lot of money on me. I guess I feel guilty. I don't want to hurt her. She's been nice to me." He looked pointedly at me. "I just don't like her as much any more. She's not like you." Yawn. Wait. What? Now, it's about this time that you're probably saying, "Give me a break." Teenage boys shouldn't be trusted and it would be unwise, Kat, for you to believe this schmuck if he tells you he wants to be with you instead of this girl. And you would be right for a number of reasons. She was eighteen just like him, while I was a sweet, young fifteen. She spent lots of money on him, while I wouldn't have access to that kind of arrangement. I mean, we did fine financially, but not extravagantly. I got paid for my work hours just like the rest of the employees. And I couldn't discount the little issue of her probably putting out to him, while I had no experience in any way at all. So while you're probably one hundred percent correct, and in agreement with my father, that I shouldn't get involved with someone who had a girlfriend like that, all I took away from the conversation was, "She's not like you."

"Well, nobody's like me," I said, in my best confident voice, with a partial sputtering quality. "And I don't think it's right to stay with someone if it's for the wrong reasons. First, it's not nice to lead her on and make her spend money..."

"Ahh, my little debater," he said, encircling me in his large, warm, and oh my, soft, yet strong arms. "That's so cute about you." So the Debate gig actually paid off, yielding romance rewards? Nice. But had he shut me up with a hug? People couldn't shut me up for anything, and believe me, they certainly tried. But I melted and it fit and I fell; completely smitten. We stayed that way for a long time, in a simple embrace. He pulled back his head and looked at me. I thought this might be it. Was his head moving closer? Eyes shutting?

Boom, boom, boom. Boom. Boom boom. The strange irregular heartbeat returned, the same as when he fell on me on the gym floor. I cleared my throat. He suddenly looked pained, almost imperceptibly shook his head and let me go. No, wait! Not yet. Don't let go yet! I'll get this heartbeat going right again in a second. But the moment had ended. I worried I'd ruined everything. So close.

But he went about flirting the rest of the shift as if nothing had changed. The following night, we ended up in an embrace again, much like the first time, only longer. It became a routine. Just the hug. I guess he thought that, if that's all there was, then no worries. He could hug me and keep his girlfriend, too. Then he started dropping me off at my house after work. That progressed to coming into my house to watch a movie, my parents long asleep, as we would arrive after midnight.

At one of our late night screenings, we sat side-by-side on the floor, with large cushions propped up behind us for comfort. I felt like Sandy from *Grease* sitting with Danny at the drive-in movie. The opening sequence to *Strange Brew* came on and we watched, ready to laugh at Canadian shtick. Then he said something to me (I don't remember what, exactly), but I had a rapid and witty retort and the next thing I knew, he tickled me. I stifled my laugh, so as not to wake the parental units, and mocked him for this obvious ruse to touch me. Before I could then call him a "hoser", he had pinned me to the floor and his lips covered mine. My heart ventured into African drumbeat territory, except with no discernible rhythm, and I had a tingling sensation all over. I kissed back but the feeling in my chest caused me great discomfort, even if no pain. Can a young girl have a heart attack or pass out from a kiss? Was this what they meant by swooning? We kissed for a while, but I couldn't enjoy it because I couldn't get my mind to shut up. Was I doing it right? Did I kiss better than Chris? Would he know this was my first time? What the bleep was going on with my heart? I rolled over, away from him, leaving him with a prime view of my tank top covered shoulder blades.

"You're not supposed to do that," he said. I think he might've been trying to help, but his whispered words only mortified me. Awkward.

"Oh, I know. I just needed to catch my breath, ya know. You kind of caught me by surprise there. Heh heh." Wow, that didn't even remotely sound like a real laugh. I took a couple of deep breaths and felt better. My heart rate slowed down and I couldn't detect the weirdness anymore. Problem hopefully averted. "I think I'm just a little tired is all. Maybe we should try this again when I'm a little more awake." He looked dejected and I wanted to slap myself. I had just rejected this person that I had pined for forever because of a pseudo heart attack. Get a grip, Kat. You're losing it, here.

I walked him to the door, my hair disheveled and my clothes slightly askew. The guilt had already taken over. Not only for my strange behavior, but for making him feel bad, and hello, for being the other woman. A home-wrecker, if that term could apply between high-school girls. I couldn't shake the feeling that I'd gotten involved in something way over my head and it frightened me. We shared one more kiss, better this time, at the door. I didn't know it at the time, but it would be our last. I had let the fears over sensations in my body destroy a momentous occasion. I won't get that back.

After that night, things changed. Of course they did. What high school guy is going to put up with that nonsense? Sensing my sudden discomfort around Nick, my dad shifted the schedule so that we hardly worked together anymore. The fun flirtation sadly ended and I was crushed like a girl in a sappy break up song. He eventually found another job. I guess the fun level really shrunk for him, too. I started avoiding the doors to his classes so that I wouldn't catch a glimpse of him in the halls. I was embarrassed. I was heartbroken. He moved on. What a shame.

What was my mind allowing to happen?

Hypochondriac Lesson #6:
Every story you hear is not a story about you.

*Chapter 6- Mad as a Hatter*

"Guess what everyone? You're in COLLEGE!"

A collective cheer erupted from the crowd of freshmen. I couldn't help but catch the contagious excitement as the orientation leaders stood in a row before us, all in matching collegiate sweatshirts, looking fresh and academic, and well, collegiate. Yes, I'd made it to college. I would no longer live at home and under the rules of my parents. I would make my own way. Change the world. Solve the problems of the planet. I had opted to begin this journey into fame, fortune, and maybe the Nobel Peace Prize, at Stetson University, a small private school in Florida, and home of the Stetson Hatters. That's right, the mascot was a hat. Most of my friends from my large public high school had matriculated to the enormous state schools but I'd decided to forge my own path and try to avoid what I imagined was little more than grade thirteen with all the people I already knew.

I'd been surprisingly ready and eager to leave the comfy nest of home and had looked at other schools out of state, but my parents could simply not afford to send me away. Times had changed for the family and things weren't quite as sunny as they'd been throughout my youth. The miniature golf business had taken a swan dive into insignificance when an unanticipated epidemic of mosquito-borne encephalitis hit the area. Or, as my father regularly referred to them, "Those damn mosquitoes." As in, "those damn mosquitoes are ruining our lives," or, "I want to kill every last one of those damn mosquitoes." Due to the sudden fear of an extremely rare disease, most of Florida from Orlando to Miami abruptly ceased venturing outdoors anytime near dusk or dawn, when mosquitoes were most prone to biting. The mosquitoes caused the school board to move football games to daylight hours, and somebody even cancelled Halloween. I'm not sure what governing body controls Halloween, but I can tell you with certainty that no kids walked the streets in costumes that night.

People panicked and the last place they wanted to entertain themselves was on a fake golf course, contending with illness breeding bloodsuckers. The air outside held the pungent scent of heavy duty insect repellent, from the general public's repeated sprays. I often wonder if evidence exists of any side effects from our potential overuse of the killer chemicals. My family's finances took a serious hit. And since we didn't fully understand the concept of financial aid for an out-of-state school, I ended up at Stetson, which had awarded me a scholarship. My parents struggled to keep their business afloat and lives somewhat manageable. They also had a new child, my baby sister Katrina, to think about. I, on the other hand, got to venture into a new phase of life and ecstatically hoped to escape the stress and melancholy. Now I would meet my new life-long best friends and start my road to international importance. Right?

After some seemingly endless icebreaker games to get to know my fellow freshmen; i.e. breaking into groups and discussing what three items we would take to a deserted island, or, and I kid you not, playing telephone; yes, the very same game we all played at say, five years of age, where we laughed uproariously, and not genuinely at all, at how a phrase changes when it travels down the line through whispered repeating; I hurried over to the bookstore to purchase my very own college sweatshirt and take ownership of my quest for knowledge. Forget walking all the way back to my dorm to change. I threw that sweatshirt right on over my boring, and so high school, solid tee shirt. There. Now I fit right in. I belonged here.

I ventured back to my new room, the furthest one from all other campus buildings. In my confusion over which school to attend, I waited too long to send a deposit and got the last choice of residence halls. The perspiration trickled down the center of my back. Perhaps I could've waited on the sweatshirt. It was still August after all. I managed to walk up the outside steps and busted in to my room, and the beautiful air conditioning, just in time to startle my new roommate in the act of hanging her clothes in the tiny indentation in the wall that served as a closet.

"Ah, there you are," I said, way too loudly; my face red and shiny from heat. "I'm Kat. It's so great to meet you." I forcibly stuck my hand out towards her. "I brought a bunch of stuff like a TV and fridge and stuff. I just wanted us to have an awesome room and you don't have to worry about getting anything really. I took care of most things." How fast was I talking? She hesitantly shook my hand.

"Well. You're enthusiastic," she said. Her voice was so deep it made me flinch unexpectedly. Then she went back to unpacking her stuff. I took in the scenery. Where was all her stuff? Did she only bring suitcases?

"Did you only bring suitcases?" I asked. I'm pretty sure it sounded like I thought she was weird.

"Yep. But like you said, you brought everything else, so…," she trailed off, facing the back of her closet so I could hardly hear her. Yeah, she was definitely weird. But I guess I needed to learn to mask my tone of voice so she wouldn't pick up on that.

"So, Darla, right?" I waited for her to respond. "'Cause that's what's on the roommate profile," I said, more to myself, since clearly she had no interest in hearing me talk. I needed to make this work. We would live together. We had to be friends. I mean, okay, so far it didn't look like we were going to be each other's bridesmaids down the road, but we needed to have at least a civil, friendly bond. I would settle for nothing less. I tried again. "It said on that sheet that I received that you play softball. That's pretty cool." She visibly perked up.

"Yeah, a bunch of girls from the team live on this hall. We were goin' to get a brewsky in a couple of minutes." She jutted her thumb in the general direction of the door, and out of feigned politeness, said, "Wanna come?" I'd never heard a female use the term "brewsky" before. And considering the noticeable deep, booming, manly nature of her voice, I might argue that I still hadn't really heard a woman say the word. I appreciated the half-hearted invitation, but decided it best to let her spend quality time with her teammates without creating even more awkward moments. I would work on our friendship once she returned.

"Oh, thanks for asking," I said in my most apologetic, gosh darn, can't-believe-I-have-to-miss-it voice. "I have so much to unpack and don't want to burden you with all my boxes in here. Plus some of my classes have already posted the first assignment, so I want to get my books and get started on that." I might've even snapped my fingers. Shucks. She shrugged, not really caring either way.

"Suit yourself."

"Yeah. Maybe next time, though?" I asked. Wow, I sounded eager.

"Mmm." Not yes, or sure, or of course. Just, mmm. Alright. So, not much luck with the roommate. College still had so much to offer, though. I was sure of it. I just didn't expect the upcoming offerings to be so bizarre.

\*\*\*

As part of my financial aid package, I had the fantastic obligation of working in the Commons; the food cafeteria, where freshmen were required to work. Due to my rigorous schedule, I could only fit my work study hours into the early morning. Granted, it was entirely self-imposed because I wanted to wade through all the required courses quickly to start learning more interesting topics. Statistics? No thanks. Let's get just that over with. Art History? Fun. Bring it on. Therefore, three days a week, I woke up at five in the morning so that I could clock in for breakfast duty at a quarter 'til six. It didn't take long to get dressed; I just had to factor in a fairly lengthy walk time. Blasted late deposit. Then I would arrive at the Commons, where I basically got to announce to the student body that I couldn't afford tuition; and mingle with the other poor kids.

There is no perfect way to describe the feeling of awesomeness that comes from walking to work in the dark, slipping on a hair net and plastic gloves to set up hot pans, and serving the food by the spoonful to your fellow students. Did you notice I mentioned a hair net? And I hadn't even turned eighteen at this point. Not a good look. I especially enjoyed changing out the hot pans over the steam trays and incurring third-degree-like burns on my fingers from the steam itself that nipped and struck at your hands and face like a transparent cobra.

"Would you like some gravy over your home fries?" I would ask through tears brought on by the constant scalding. Luckily, the students couldn't really see me crying through the foggy sneeze guard.

While my experience working there provided lots of "fun" and "memorable" times, my personal favorite Commons moment arrived one day when the shift manager, always an upper-classman who wanted extra money but didn't want to work that hard, got angry because I dropped a tray (an extremely hot tray, I might add; skin-blisteringly hot) of bacon on the floor, creating a loss for the food service team. As my punishment, she placed me on waffle duty. Doesn't sound so bad, right? I mean, yum, waffles are tasty. But have you ever used a commercial-grade waffle iron and know offhand the perfect level of batter necessary to make one Belgian Waffle? No? Neither did the students at Stetson University. I would stand nearby, as I was not actually supposed to make the waffles, and watch. And wait. Which meant that me and my hair net were no longer protected by any barriers from view. I was on full display for the destruction. In the entire year that

I worked there, I never once saw a person use the waffle iron without making at least a small mess. Most messes, though, were more in the nature of a volcanic eruption where the batter oozed like lava all over the counter, into the waffle toppings, down the cabinet walls and, if I was lucky, spread onto the floor in a thick, custard-colored lake.

I watched each student struggle with the waffle iron, and provided assistance when I could; usually only if they came alone, since I found it impossible to break up a group conversation with waffling instructions. I used my disgusting, wet, gray rag to wipe up the viscous substance after each use, then would retreat to rinse it out, watching about a pound of batter hit the bottom of the sink at each cleaning. Then back out to the floor. Well, after one rinsing, I had apparently missed quite a doozy. I saw the back of the guy as he headed to the register with his waffle but quickly turned to the doughy massacre that had preceded his edible creation. He must've used all the batter in the bucket because it slid, and pooled and drained just about anywhere the eye could see. Shift Manager rushed to my side.

"Where have you been?" she asked, hissing like a viper. "How could you let it get this messy?"

"I'm so sorry," I said, "I just went to rinse out my rag."

"Well this is terrible! Let me go see if there's someone else I can send out here to help you get this up." I hurriedly tried to clean up the culinary catastrophe. I couldn't afford to lose this job; it would mean I couldn't afford school. In my rush to mop up the goop, I didn't see that I'd stepped into some stray batter. I lost my footing, and suddenly found myself clinging to the side of the counter (good reflexes, if I do say so myself), while my feet did a rapid sliding dance of their own, as if ice skating, threatening to send me into a split. The rag in my hand didn't allow me to have a strong enough grip on the counter's edge and I rapidly discovered myself on my back, writhing on the floor, causing the batter to cover more surface area of my body than necessary. I immediately felt like the Karate Kid, when he falls in the spaghetti at the country club while spying on his beloved. I heard laughing, snickering, whispering, but I didn't hear any offer of assistance. In fact, when I managed to focus for a split second on the world around me, I noticed that people were definitely watching, but not really sure what to do. I let out a sharp noise, somewhere in the middle of a yelp and a grunt. Finally, Shift Manager stomped over to me in a huff. She managed to pull me up even though my slippery feet protested, and together we straightened up the area. The rest of the cafeteria resumed normal behavior but my embarrassment overwhelmed me. None of these people would bust walls to befriend me. The only bright spot was that due to my demonstrated incompetence, Shift Manager didn't put me on the waffle station anymore, and I could continue to exist with the comfort of hair net anonymity and scorched appendages behind the counter.

I ended up lonely and sad at college. I hadn't signed up for this. I'd expected parties and "Animal House" and life-changing friendships, and sitting under a tree with a professor and group of students talking about philosophy. Not hair nets and five a.m. scaldings. Not manly roommates that think you're ridiculous for not grabbing a brewsky. I ate alone. I would arrive for work and the shift manager would send each employee out to eat breakfast for fifteen minutes. I ate those dastardly waffles. Hey, they created enough problems, might as well enjoy some of the benefits. Or I ate biscuits with gravy, or scrambled eggs with bacon and home fries. Truth be told, the food was not awful. In an effort to avoid eating solo in the cafeteria during the busy lunch hour when everyone arrives in friend clusters, I opted to get take-out at the campus café; fried cheese sticks, or chicken strips with honey mustard. For dinner, I would do the same, or I would order a pizza delivered to my dorm room for solitary consumption. Somehow, eating alone, it's easy to consume more quantities. So it will come as no surprise that I gained the freshmen fifteen with quite a bit of ease. Depression will do that to a gal.

In the meantime, while I struggled to make a connection with my school and the other students, my parents struggled with their own issues. They realized that they could do little to turn their business around and made the hard decision to close the doors. The stress took its toll and the doctors told my father that he had high blood pressure. Now, honestly, this news didn't shock or even surprise me, or anyone who knew my father in the slightest. My father had always excelled as a bit of a "screamer." He and I rarely discussed. Instead, we just yelled at each other. He tended to exude high levels of Sam Kinison stress on most occasions. My mother often joked that with his constant dramatics and histrionic reactions to issues, he was "trying to win an Oscar." As in, "Oh the batteries on the remote went dead while your dad was watching Perry Mason and we didn't have extras and now he's trying to win an Oscar." Friends, relatives and random strangers predicted my father would have a heart attack one day. For the doctor to mention to my dad that he should try to calm down really didn't offer any new realizations.

"The doctor also said your dad's cholesterol is high," said my mom. "He needs to try to eat better."

At the time, my family didn't know as much about the causes of heart disease as we unfortunately do now, so the idea that the foods that we ate could have ill effects on our bodies didn't register clearly.

"He said that he could have a heart attack if he doesn't get it together."

"So, like, what does he need to change?" I asked while eating a potato skin at a local restaurant. My parents, noting that school and my lack of friends made me blue, kindly drove the half hour to take me to dinner a couple of times a week.

They didn't like the idea that I ate by myself all the time; although in hindsight, this was probably not the best way for them to spend their limited resources, nor the best way to improve their diets.

"I think he just needs to cut down on red meat, fried foods, and butter. Things like that. The doctor said something about cheese as well." I looked down at my fried potato skin with cheese sauce (was that even real cheese?) and set it down, slightly unnerved.

"He shouldn't eat cheese?" I'd eaten nothing but cheese, practically. I may not eat burgers all the time, but cheese? I consumed cheese like breathing oxygen. Then I started to think about the other foods I ate frequently. Fried, fatty, sweet. Oh no. Let's face it, even I knew that nobody should eat country gravy on a daily basis. Yet I tossed those thickly drenched biscuits back like I would waste away otherwise. I had set myself up for the same thing as my father. But wait. It's okay. He hadn't actually had a heart attack. This was just a warning. The doctor said this just to try to start my dad onto the good habits, right?

"The doctor said that the first step to getting healthier is to lose some weight. Being overweight can vastly increase chances for high blood pressure and high cholesterol."

I felt like I might throw up the smothered tuber that I'd just consumed. What had I done? In my misery, I'd taken the same course as my parents. I'd eaten all the wrong things and now I, too, would get high cholesterol and probably have a heart attack. The stress of school and my current social failures would raise my blood pressure. Oh mercy. Did I even know the whereabouts of the local hospital? I hoped it was close, just in case. My dad licked the sauce off his fingers as he finished the last rib on his plate.

"I'll be fine. I just won't eat as many hamburgers." Somehow I didn't think that getting healthy would arrive simply for any of us. But I had to take the challenge.

\*\*\*

Over the next several weeks, I went about my business with the inspirational "Rocky" anthem in my head; the one that plays when he's training and you know it will make all the difference in the world against his adversary, Mr. T, or that big Russian guy. I started to cut back on the size of my meals. I didn't eat as much fried food. I said a few heartbreaking goodbyes to cheese; like young lovers separated by war. I tried to pick up my pace a little as I walked around campus. The doctor's words to my father had shaken me. I was fairly certain that I already had high numbers in both the blood pressure and cholesterol categories, but since a test for cholesterol levels requires a needle, I opted for a lifestyle change and just hoped for the best. I can't say I had an easy time. On a chilly morning, biscuits and gravy can tempt a little more easily than a fruit plate. The angel and devil on my shoulders fought a lot. I cannot claim perfection. But as I ate the gravy, I started to develop the idea that I could actually feel the dense fluid/solid clogging my arteries and corroding my veins. When this thought popped into my mind, I couldn't get past it and would lower my fork in disgust. I lost ten pounds. For once I had a little control over my fears. I had taken action. I felt empowered by my worries. Now if only I could make some friends.

A peculiar group of events soon occurred that pushed me towards contemplating some important decisions about my college career. The first episode came in the classroom. I sat beside a guy in my intro history course named John. He engaged me with a pleasant demeanor, speaking to me at each class, which I relished since I had so little interaction otherwise. He always wanted to discuss the topics of the day with me. Maybe I'd finally found the academic discourse I'd so eagerly craved. Then one day the professor approached me, quietly taking me aside. In a low voice, he asked me if I would mind tutoring John as he had had some trouble turning a couple of papers in for grades.

"The work I've seen has been, how should I say this, subpar," said the professor. No problem. I would love to help. This would mean more human conversation outside of class. Hurrah. I told John to meet me and we could go over his papers.

At the campus café, he handed me three papers. And I mean exactly what I've said. The professor had assigned us three papers; eight to ten typed pages each, double-spaced. John handed me three sheets of wide-ruled notebook paper, each representing the three individual assignments. On each page he had written his sentences in all capital letters like a serial killer, had skipped a line in between each row (this must have been his interpretation of the double-spacing requirement) and had zero punctuation. As if this wasn't enough, he appeared to have a strong aversion to subject-verb agreement. For example, John might have written, "the elephant ate three peanut" had the topic revolved around circuses. None of these practices worked particularly well for a history paper. I had no clue where to start.

"Is this an outline?" I asked, trying to mask my disbelief and give him the benefit of the doubt.

"No," he said, then turned his head in shame.

I felt bad, but didn't he have to write an essay to even get into the school? This did not equate to what I had in mind for stimulating intellectual discourse. I know plenty of smart students must have attended that school, but given my limited connectivity to any of them, I suddenly felt concerned for my own academic progression, if my peers were people at John's level. Maybe I should think about transferring. Would I have better luck at another school? I didn't want my mind to turn into sludge. I had enough to worry about with my body deteriorating.

The second episode confirmed my suspicion that I needed to make a clean break. I woke early each morning, frustrated. I was mad that I had to wake up with the chickens to work in a hot kitchen. I grew agitated that I didn't learn what I wanted to learn in school; ticked that I had failed to surround myself with the academic elite. On one morning, I trudged down to the hall bathroom, shared by all thirty people on the floor, in my fuzzy slippers, a vision of fatigue and defeat. The overhead fluorescent lights of the bathroom cast a pall over my face and I shivered. I opened the door to a stall and stood there for a while, trying to process my view. In the toilet rested three oranges. Bright orange. Not rotten. I blinked a few times. I must be tired. Is there citrus in the toilet? After a while, I turned back to the mirror and stared at myself. Who would even bring citrus into the bathroom? That's a tad on the gross side. And then, how does it come about that three whole pieces of fruit end up in the commode? I puzzled over this for quite some time. I almost had to run for work, late.

The next morning my visit to the bathroom provided a new mystery with popcorn in all six sinks, and oh, yes, there it is, in two toilets, as well. Again I considered the possibilities. I could see bringing in a dirty popcorn bowl to wash out. But there was no microwave in the bathroom. Students did not have the opportunity to cook and/or store food in the lavatory, so why would anyone bring this much popcorn into the bathroom. It really was a significant amount. I'm talking large-tub-at-the-movie-theatre size. Then once in the bathroom, how or why does one disburse the kernels into all open vessels? Does the culprit confuse the sinks and toilets with trash cans? Perhaps in a panicked state, the person desperately wants to find a garbage disposal, tries each sink, then discovering that none of them have one, decides that a toilet is the next best thing? Very curious incidences indeed. I could hardly think of anything else on the days when I would find these little brainteasers. For once, I could put into practice all that I'd learned from those sleuthing TV lawyers I so adored.

The "popcorn perplexity," as I had named the occurrences, happened on several occasions, making the original discovery even more troubling, because then I couldn't logically blame it on inebriation. Do drunk people do the same strange actions multiple times on different occasions? If that's the case, then they seriously needed to think about expanding their repertoire. And the perp completely blew my theories out of the water (no pun intended) when I discovered popcorn and an apple in the shower. Were they so hungry that they couldn't even bathe without a snack? All hail the almighty shower shoes. Best two dollars I ever spent. Wet food doesn't seem like a good idea for bare feet. The sanitation issues were eating away at me, like the culprit of all these snacks.

One morning I woke up even earlier than usual. My Shift Manager at the Commons had asked me to come in for a special event set up, so my alarm horrifyingly went off at a quarter to five. I yawned, blindly stuffed my feet into my slippers, wrapped my robe around me, grabbed my plastic portable shower caddy and ventured quietly out the door so as not to wake an irritated Darla. Our relationship hadn't improved and I hadn't been asked out for another brewsky. About halfway down the hallway I came upon a mound. I didn't have my glasses on so I walked nearer, but slowly, always hesitant of the unknown. The mound looked misshapen and dark brown. I squinted as I got closer and, no, it couldn't be. Piled in front of my eyes, in a college dorm, at a University costing over twenty grand a year, lay a steaming pile of human feces. What the hell (a "bleep" simply wouldn't cut it in this case)? I started my usual Sherlock Holmes internal questioning, but couldn't get over the basic one. What would possess a semi-intelligent person, a girl, no less; as this was a strict girls-only dorm; to remove her pants and defecate right in the middle of a hallway shared by thirty other girls, when the bathroom is only another fifteen feet away?

I would never receive an answer to my multiple queries. But these events coupled with my ongoing "death by cholesterol" anxiety caused me to evaluate my current existence. Between the strange insanity at school and my parents' sad and worrisome circumstances in both health and finances, I needed to escape as fast as possible. I craved the chance to embrace a new life. Hopefully feces free in shared spaces. Time to transfer.

Hypochondriac Lesson #7:
Do not self-diagnose unless you have a medical degree.

### 7- One Isn't So Lonely a Number When There are Onlookers

Ahhh. Now this is what I'm talking about. The bell from the tower rings on the hour, currently the eight o'clock hour; early morning to some, but decadently late to me. It sounds like fairies sprinkling magic into the lobes of my brain. I inhale and smell flowers and trees, honeysuckles and magnolias, slightly wet from the morning mist. My feet land softly on the beautifully old stone pathways and I watch the morning veil lift as the sun permeates through the thick blanket of leaves. I feel like I might have reached heaven on earth, although I doubt in heaven I'll wear a flannel shirt. I peer around at the students walking to class, looking as if they materialized out of the pages of a J. Crew catalog, and I realize I might need to up the ante on my wardrobe a bit. But such is life at my new college home, Vanderbilt University.

The transfer process had a few bumps and dips along the way. After securing my place in the Vandy Class of 1997, and convincing them of my worth for a near full scholarship, my parents discovered that they didn't really have the means to drop me off and move me into the school. So I solicited the help of an old high school friend and his truck, and together we drove the eleven hours to get me there in time for orientation. The poor guy then turned around, after lugging all my heavy boxes around, and drove the entire way back home. I feel like that guy deserves an annual thank you; at least a Christmas card. Not many people are that nice. Meanwhile, the incoming class count had reached an all-time high that year, which left a shortage of housing. The R.A. of the dorm showed me to my room, a delightfully converted study lounge with bunk beds plunked down haphazardly. Four of us would share this room until they could find an alternative housing solution for us.

"I promise this isn't permanent," the R. A. assured us, nervous and slightly sweaty. He eagerly and sweetly desired to make us as comfortable as possible for such an inconvenience. You could see that the stress had trickled down from the housing office. We could imagine administrators yelling, "Students pay over thirty grand a year to go here, make sure they understand that we will fix this."

But we, the three other transfers and me, fluttered with joy from leaving our respective previous schools. We actually enjoyed living together and considered it more like bliss than a hindrance. We just had to remember to keep the swinging double doors locked, because not everyone in the building understood that students currently lived in those study lounges. I can't even count on both hands the number of times I would sit on my bed, engaged in a little class reading, perhaps an afternoon of light Nietzsche, when the door would swing open, someone would enter, not paying attention, then suddenly realize something was off.

"What the hell? Why are there beds in here?" Then he or she or they would make eye contact with me, looking like an animal caught in headlights, and say, "Oh shit, I'm so sorry." Then they would arch backward to look at the outside of the door again, as if asking themselves if they were that out of it that they would randomly walk into someone's dorm room. Seeing the plaque indicating "study lounge," the confusion only escalated and they couldn't accept it, or wouldn't accept it.

"This IS the study lounge, right?"

"Yep."

"So are you just in here studying?" They would look around, noticing stuff like makeup and shampoo caddies, fluffy slippers and framed photos of strangers. Yet they remained fully ready to embrace the place as their temporary study habitat. I couldn't help but laugh, until they looked stricken. I would clear my face.

"I'm sorry, I should've locked the door. This is actually a temporary dorm room until they can place us in better housing."

"Oh," they would say, relieved that they weren't the crazy ones. Then, "That sucks for you." Every time. I heard it on a daily basis. No, I wanted to say, let me tell you about some stuff that sucks for me. This place is definitely not one of them.

In under three weeks, the school kept their promise and placed all four of us into permanent housing. Unfortunately, they spread us apart to such a degree that it proved difficult to socialize as often now that we busily tried to acclimate to our coursework and various activities. Transferring can be difficult if most of your credits won't transfer with you. I had taken a class on Welsh at Stetson. Only a small percentage of the population of Wales even speaks Welsh these days, but now I have some of that information in my head forever; not terribly useful, and not something that transfers to other schools. So typically, as a transfer, you have to kill yourself with your course load if you want to graduate on time. And killing myself led me down the road to some health issues.

I had ended up with a single room on a hall with a shared bathroom in an upper classman all-girls dorm. I loved the fabulous location, a picturesque brick building with stone accents sitting right on the main lawn; the centerpiece of campus. My favorite feature was the campus bell tower visible above the trees in the distance. But as I got to know the other ladies on the hall, I couldn't help but wonder if they had chosen to live in these singles more because they were serious about their studies and didn't want any distractions, or because they had difficult cohabitation problems, and couldn't find a roommate brave enough to take the plunge of sharing space.

My favorite of the singles dwellers on my floor was a girl by the name of The Tactless One. Now clearly, this wasn't her real name. I cannot actually remember her first name. I remember it as something like Carrie, or Jenny, or Marcie maybe. I'm not sure I ever even called her by her first name. I said something like, "Hey there. You." This kind of makes me sound like the tactless one. But in my own mind or when I would share stories about her to others (not that I make a habit of talking about people behind their backs, mind you), I always referred to her as The Tactless One. And here's why.

As you might have guessed, the girl had no tact whatsoever. But it was not your run-of-the-mill lack of tact. She took it to clinically significant levels. She would say things like, "These oranges are rotten and don't taste good. Do you want them?" Let me see. You won't eat them because they will make you sick. Please, let me at 'em. Can't wait. Or, on another occasion she casually asked me if I had any formal dresses with me at school. I replied that I had indeed brought a couple of formals with me. At that point, I hadn't made up my mind about sororities and was keeping my options open. Plus I always harbored illusions of having formal dates in college. Vanderbilt was a good place in that regard; full of southern charm and traditions. Then she asked me what size I wore. What size were those formal dresses?

I looked in my closet. "They're a size four."

"Hmm. I'm not sure if that'll work or not," she replied.

"Why? What are you asking for?"

"Well Erica needs to go to a formal. She doesn't have a date yet, but she thinks she will by the end of the week. And she doesn't have a dress to wear. I thought if you have one, maybe she could borrow yours."

"Wait, YOUR friend Erica? The engineering major?" I asked. She nodded in the affirmative and my mouth dropped.

You see, I'm about 5'5" and my dresses, as noted, were a size four. After my initial freshman year problem with weight gain, I had slimmed back down to my high school fighting weight. Erica, on the other hand, stood not quite five feet tall. And I don't want to be mean here but she was, how should I put it, not currently a size four. In fact I would wager on more like a size sixteen. Which is fine. Everybody has a different body type. My problem with the situation was that the Tactless One seemed to think that my body type was the same as Erica's. And nobody likes to hear that they look as if they are multiple sizes bigger than their actual size. It's unpleasant and in this case, rather shocking. This was a fairly clear case.

"Umm, no," I said, tactfully, in direct contrast to my now-nemesis, "I don't think that will work." I paused. "But I hope Erica finds something that will suit her." The Tactless One just shrugged, almost like a bored "whatever." The nerve of that girl.

I later shared this story with my friend Mike, another Engineering student who knew both the Tactless One and Erica from his classes. Also, unbeknownst to him, he was the object of Erica's affection and intended date target for the formal in question. He started laughing wildly and said, "I can't believe she asked you that. Are you kidding me? You could grease Erica up with Crisco and give her a running start and she STILL wouldn't be able to fit into your dress. If you want your dress to remain in one piece, that is." Ouch. He held his stomach as he cackled. "But wait, maybe she wanted to know if you had a couple, then they could patch them all together to make one dress!" His laugh grew maniacal. Double ouch. Luckily Erica never built up the nerve to ask Mike. That would have ended ugly. I just hope that the Tactless One didn't go back to Erica and say something like, "Oh Kat had some dresses, but they never would've fit you in a million years." I would wager she said something equally offensive.

I tried to avoid her as much as possible. It was hard because she lived only a few feet away and everybody needs a study break. But my classes and work study schedule kept me relatively busy so that I only really had the pleasure of her company sometimes at night, if we both faced a long evening of studying in our rooms. Even then, if I knew for sure that she would be in her room, I would make a point to find another place to study.

It was after a late night of studying away from my room, at a study lounge in the student center, that the "Absurdist Gerald Ford Incident" occurred. Facing an all-nighter of reading and paper writing, I indulged in not one, but four Mountain Dews. The sweet, horribly yellow, highly caffeinated beverage infused my cells and gave me a jolt, helping me rapidly wade through the work, keeping me going through the dark, chilly hours of the early morning, and enabling me to complete all my assignments. I stumbled into my room around five a.m. and collapsed into my bed, my eyes blurry and unable to see much of my surroundings.

At seven a.m. my alarm went off. I sat up and thought I might puke at the same time. I ran my tongue around the inside of my mouth. It tasted of chemical and had a film of sticky, mucous-like goo on my palette. Ick. Also, my bed felt like it vibrated, like one of those nasty hotel beds you can put coins into the slot to make it shake. Then, I realized it might be me vibrating and not the bed. I wiped my forehead and noted the sweat creating a slick line on my finger where it had touched my skin. Oookay. It wasn't really that hot in here. I swung my legs over the side of my bed, stood up, and sat right back down. So dizzy. What was going on? I instinctively put my hand up to my chest and felt the rapid flutter of my heart rather than the steady beat that I normally felt. Uh oh. This could not be good. I can hear you say, well, it was the caffeine. And while this would logically explain my feelings, I had no idea of that at the time. I had never consumed caffeine like that before and had no idea of the effects it would bring. I never drank coffee. I thought it tasted like tar, or what I imagined tar to taste like, and while growing up, my family only drank decaffeinated sodas and teas. Mostly I drank water. I was in no way prepared for the onslaught of physicality that my caffeine consumption created. But I had dragged sluggishly the previous day, and Mike had casually suggested that I either take a No Doze or I should drink some Mountain Dew. I was opposed completely to the No Doze. I would not take a pill to get homework done. I had seen enough "after-school specials" and an episode of "Saved By the Bell" that kept me in line on that front. So I opted for the Mountain Dew. I thought it would help keep me awake, not send me into outer space.

I shakily put on my bathrobe, weakly grabbed my shower caddie and headed down to the bathroom. The water of the shower helped me regroup a little but the drops felt like electricity on my skin. Could I be having a seizure of some sort? I dropped my razor six times as I tried to shave my legs; my fingers just couldn't seem to keep their grip on the handle. Maybe I had early onset Parkinson's. I flinched as I cut myself on the leg and watched the droplets of blood sink through the drain. I held my hands up in front of my face in the shower and observed as they twitched, moving even though my brain tried to tell them to stop. That's it. I definitely had Parkinson's. I leaned my head back to quickly rinse my hair so I could finish up in here and give myself time before class to stop by the library and see if I could find any information about the disease. I know I was tired, but fatigue never caused me to shake like this. My whole body buzzed from the inside out. When I brought my head back up, a wave of vertigo enveloped me and I had to use my quaking hands to find security against the wall. Oooh. Wish I hadn't touched the wall like that. Okay, better get out of the shower, before I pass out and someone gets to be the lucky person who finds a shaking naked girl on the floor of a hall shower. Fun for all involved.

Back in my room, I carefully got dressed. After an initial failure trying to button up a shirt, I tossed it to the ground and opted for a plain tee shirt. Fashion held importance, but in my current state, I felt lucky to have the ability to put the clothes on, so coverage had to take precedent. I reached for my deodorant. Where was my deodorant? It always sat right on the end of my chest of drawers, right next to my hair spray, adjacent to my curling iron. This never changes. Considering the size of the room was little more than a glorified closet, not a lot of other locations existed in which to store such necessities. I looked around frantically; not helping the dizziness. Great. I had to run and take a French test. I was nervous, would probably sweat and now officially had lost my deodorant. Is that something that people even lose? I quickly rooted around the room in a last attempt to find the stick of good hygiene or anything else that might work in its place. My hand rested on a box at the bottom of my closet that I simply referred to as "my miscellaneous box," a hodgepodge of extras that existed for the entire time I lived at the University, but I only ever used this once. I don't ever remember assembling this box, but the contents seemed to change. It held recipes and chocolate and incense and a brush and paper clips and a package of instant grits. Today in the box I found a bottle of body powder.

I have never in my life used body powder. I choose deodorant, a spray or two of perfume. Even smelly lotions had a momentary role in my life; but never body powder. I wasn't even a hundred percent sure where to put it. I don't know where I got it. It came in a metal bottle and looked kind of fancy and very floral.

I could either smell like nervous perspiration, or I could puff this under my arms and smell, temporarily at least, like an English Garden. I sprinkled a mound into my hand and smeared it onto my armpit, then reversed hands and did it to the other side. The dust covered my hands and residue had drifted onto the jeans I had already put on. A good look, made worse when I made an effort to clear the specks off the pants. I smacked my hands together to clean them off and coughed as the air turned cloudy and aromatic around my face. This stuff was strong. And certainly understanding that the powder would likely not work very well as an antiperspirant (I was already so hot and moist), I could only hope that my armpits wouldn't make a substance like paste, and create tell-tale goopiness on my clothes. I had no time to ponder the possibilities further and had to hope for the best. Perhaps I should not have put so much on, though. I sneezed a rapid four times in a row as I left my room and headed out across campus.

I started strong out the door but after about fifty feet, I felt like my body hit a wall. My backpack weighed so much. How was it possible that I had carried this thing in the past? It seemed like only a weight lifter could possibly have the strength. My body continued to vibrate but felt heavy at the same time. I was pretty sure I would need to stop and throw up into the bushes. I'm sure the landscaping team would thoroughly frown on puke in their tulips, so I tried my best to focus on reaching my destination. Then I heard the buzzing. It was at first distant sounding and I was fairly certain that it came from inside my body. I mean, if I felt the buzzing it stood to reason that I would hear it, too, right? But then the buzzing moved closer and the volume rose in my ear. The visual caught up with the audio. A bee! No wait. Two bees! Buzzing around me, doing as nature intended for them to do, find the flower.

By this point my jelly feet had allowed me to travel up to the main epicenter of student activity and crowds. Alone and in plain sight of a large portion of campus, I had no choice but to try to fight the bees. One had landed on my shoulder while the other flew menacingly around my head. I swatted them away, difficult considering my arm had the weight of a bag of sand. I would keep walking. Maybe the swat would do the trick. No, that was not to be. Instead they swarmed back (if two can swarm) with intense fury, this time both landing on my shoulder, in an effort to find the mysterious hidden garden in my armpit. As I swatted them both away a second time, going against all my mother ever taught me about not making bees mad, one bee decided it had had enough of my aggressiveness and zipped around to my other arm, casually injecting that dastardly, and painful, little stinger into my arm. Ha. Gotcha garden woman.

I shrieked and started to slap at myself frantically. The bees had my focus at shoulder height and I paid no attention to where my still-moving feet carried me. Until, that is, I noticed for a split second that my foot had not landed where it should on level concrete and I tumbled, head over backpack over feet, down the three steps that led from the student union walkway onto a sidewalk towards my intended classroom building. I crumpled there, contorted, not sure what to do first. My arm killed me. I definitely needed to get that checked out. I didn't think anything had broken. A tall guy with glasses came up to me, concerned, and helped to pull my compromised body up off the ground. I assured him I was fine and didn't need an escort to Student Health, even though I wasn't quite so sure about this. I heard the bell tower chime its sweet melody and realized that my French test started right now. I waved at the nice stranger, who was so much better than the mean laughers at the Stetson University Commons, and did my best impression of hurrying to my class.

By the time I got to the building, the crowds had cleared, as everyone now sat comfortably seated in class or headed back to their dorm rooms for a nap. The elevator was out of order, of course, so I started my trek up the four flights of stairs. By the second flight, all my remaining adrenaline drain. My body crashed. I didn't have the energy to make the rest of the steps. I was sure of it. The bee sting, well, stung like crazy. It had puffed, red and swollen. Great. Now I had Parkinson's and some terrible allergic reaction to bees. I waited for my throat to close up. I took the next step, tripped and fell flat out on the stairs, by body complimenting the angle of the staircase perfectly, like a cartoon character. I gave up. My back pack weighed on me, just too heavy, pressing me flatter against the steps. I just stayed there for a while.

When I later told Mike about the episode, he said, "Why do you fall all the time? You're like that Chevy Chase skit about Gerald Ford on Saturday Night Live. Except the circumstances that make you fall are so absurd. I mean, who falls because of bees and caffeine crashes? Or waffle irons?" Absurdist Gerald Ford. A nickname from Mike. So there you go.

After convincing the French teacher to allow me to make up my test on a better day when I didn't need medical attention, I visited Student Health. I cried as they tended to the sting, not because it hurt, but because I really thought something had gone wrong with me. Why did I shake and fall and get dizzy? I was terrified. The doctor asked about my activities during the last twenty-four hours, then laughed at me. It wouldn't be the last time a doctor would laugh at me, but I can tell you I did not enjoy it.

"I suggest you stay off caffeine." He chuckled heartily. "It doesn't seem to be very good for your system. Put that together with lack of sleep and stress and you have a bit of a problem. Maybe you should try to get your work done during normal hours when you don't have to supplement your body's natural ability to stay awake." That was pretty good advice. Still, I'd never seen anyone else respond to caffeine like this. Did that mean that I had some underlying problem. I, of course, asked him as such.

"No. You're just not used to caffeine, and the quantity and circumstances of your little adventure were just less tolerated by your body. Please try not to worry." Right. Easier said than done. He gave me a large cup of water and told me to stay well hydrated and sent me back to my dorm.

As I entered the dorm and headed to my room, I noticed that The Tactless One had her door open, so I thought I would peek my head in and tell her of my morning insanity. As I regaled her with the tale, my eyes hit upon something strange on her desk. My deodorant. No, it can't be. You may ask, "Kat, how do you really know it was your deodorant? People often use the same brand, yes?" Ah, but you see, out of boredom one day while I took a break from studying and watched a little *Days Of Our Lives* on my teeny tiny TV, I had taken a black Sharpie and doodled on my deodorant casing. A smiley face, a child-like sunshine, and a flower, which is a little ironic for this tale. And there, on her desk, the same doodles on the same stick. She saw my eyes drift over to the stick. I saw her eyes see my eyes. There was now no mistaking that we both knew what was going on. But I just kept talking, animated about my bee incident. I clearly didn't want the deodorant back. And if she needed some so much that she had to steal it, well then, I guess she could just have it. I would get more. As if having early Parkinson's wasn't enough, I had to deal with a thief in the mix; one that lived up to her well-earned nickname.

Hypochondriac Lesson#8:
If you have nothing in common with a victim,
chances are you don't have the same disease.

## 8- "Hello, My Name is Kat. How Can I Help You?"

"Did you find everything you needed today?" I asked the gentleman, in the same tone I had used approximately eighty-seven other times that afternoon. I slid each of his items across the scanner.

"Oh, I found everything I need," he said. He made a strange and lascivious expression, licking his lips. He eyed the contents of his hand-held grocery basket, and then met my eyes knowingly as I continued to glide each item across the counter absentmindedly. I hardly ever registered what people bought. Usually, I just stayed in my own thoughts and went through the motions. But this time I decided to take notice since he seemed so keen to point out his purchases. Steak, red wine, bread, condoms. Well, okay then. Guy was apparently pretty proud of the fact that he thought he would get lucky tonight. I wanted to suggest that he might consider a side dish to up his chances, but what did I know? Do women find just steak on a plate the pinnacle of romance? I don't. How about a nice side salad, at least? All in all, his gross voice and dirty eye contact seemed like a little too much information for the local cashier.

That's right folks. While other students from my most esteemed university spent their summers glamorously interning in New York City, or studying abroad in exotic locales, or just working at the beach somewhere, I whiled away the hours of this summer after sophomore year earning slightly more than minimum wage as a cashier at a grocery store. I had the pleasure of wearing the most "attractive" ensemble of pastel polyester you could ever imagine. The fabric of my sea foam green vest looked and felt flammable. The peach bowtie added a whimsical je ne sais quoi to my short-sleeved white button down shirt. Add on the crazy flattering navy blue pleated pants and I had a look that could stop traffic. The fashion elite might as well have put me straight on the catwalk in Paris. I contemplated telling

my employers that my nickname was "Charlie" or "Donna," so that my nametag

would not forever connect my actual name with this vision of loveliness.

I must take a moment to digress and acknowledge that my job and outfit

as a cashier of the local grocery store didn't actually count as the worst job I'd

ever had. In fact, that accolade went to my job from the previous summer after

my freshman year at Stetson. As if the year hadn't afforded me enough misery,

I took the only job that would give me full time work. Bmart. I held the highly

regarded, by no one, title of "Fashion Customer Service Associate." I think you

should read that title again. At Bmart. Before any famous people started creating

clothing lines for the discount stores. I wore a red polyester smock. I stocked sock

packages, mysteriously destroyed less than fifteen minutes later, even if nobody

had come through to buy socks. I got berated regularly by angst ridden customers

irritated by our lack of size diversity of the Wranglers on sale that week. On

really exceptional days, the bosses appointed me to watch the jewelry counter

while Jewelry Manager went on her lunch hour. This was nerve wracking and did

nothing to help my growing general anxiety. Jewelry Manager had not properly

trained me on jewelry repair and maintenance; or even the register. I accidentally

sold a two hundred dollar gold bracelet for $14.99, although, if you ask me, the

grotesque rope of gold wasn't worth a penny more. I also broke a watch band,

and shattered the glass of a watch face, when a person brought their watch in for

a simple battery change. I created that much Bmart jewelry mayhem all in one

day. When Jewelry Manager discovered my mistake in the fine jewelry sale, she

shrugged and said in a thick smoker's voice, "Well at least they paid you something

for it. Most of the time they just try to steal things." Nice. The reality of the

situation was that Grocery Store Cashier was like a glorious and relaxing vacation compared to duties in discount "fashion."

In some ways, I felt lucky. I didn't have to face people that I knew. My family now lived in Georgia in a busy suburb outside of Atlanta. They had left Florida in an attempt to escape the stigma of financial failure. Once their business faltered, they had to shut the doors, and endured foreclosure on the house where I grew up. They couldn't face their friends, and worse, the community of endless acquaintances who would really talk. My mother started shopping at a grocery store twenty miles away so that she wouldn't run into anyone when she used her food stamps. Things had gotten pretty tough, so they fled; physically and emotionally. Now they lived in a duplex in a subsidized community, after staying for a couple of weeks with some old friends in the area. My parents said they wanted to start fresh. The silver lining I found in all of this was that after working at Bmart in my old neighborhood, where I had once been considered well off and slightly spoiled, I could now enjoy the comfort of my polyester vest without worry that anyone I had known my entire life would see me.

Most of the time, my shift went by as fast as microwavable food. I could guess the amount of time that had passed based on the number of orders I'd processed. Baskets brimming with food could take north of five minutes. More if I had to bag the groceries myself. And while I never committed the cardinal sin of squashing bread with canned food, or anything like that, I hardly considered myself a bagging expert. I tended to make some bags too heavy and others too light, resulting in customers with lopsided discomfort as they attempted to exit the store. And if a person wrote a check, well, then we faced double the time, at least. Smaller orders, such as steak-on-a-plate-I'm-gonna-get-busy-tonight guy, I tried to push through in under a minute. It was a race. With myself. And I was the only one who cared. But I had to do something to make it interesting.

During slow times I stood out in front of my line and asked weary looking shoppers if they were ready to check out as they passed by me. Even if they weren't heading towards the front, my manager insisted I ask them if I could help them make their purchase. I found this strange. Typically in a grocery store when shoppers finish, they know where to head. You never see someone standing in the back corner of the store looking worried and frustrated because they don't know what to do now that they've found their food. I guess the manager just wanted to make sure we spoke to the lowest common denominator. Fine. But I also thought the request peculiar because wasn't the object of the grocery store business to have the customer spend as much money as possible? If we rushed them through, they wouldn't have the opportunity for the Twinkie impulse buy, or the pie that wasn't on the list but just looked good. I pondered these things as I verbally attacked, in a professional and friendly way, each customer who walked by.

"I can check you out right here, if you're ready." Startled look to me, followed by an unsure look into their basket.

"Uh...no, thanks...I have a few more things to get."

"Okay," I would reply, all smiles and snap-gun hands. "Let me know if I can help you." Even though I got a similar response each time, I harbored an idea that the managers watched on the security cameras and knew if I didn't speak to every person who crossed my path. I never was much of a rule breaker. But I did take the time, when no patrons lurked on the horizon, to peruse the covers of the latest magazines. I felt never so bold to take one off the shelf and shuffle through the pages. But I had a pretty good handle on tabloid headlines. I knew generally which recent celebrity had a nose job, or who couldn't seem to control their cellulite on the beach. Weight loss, weight gain, divorce, marriage, UFO sightings; all eye candy during a slow afternoon. Then I saw one that literally took my breath away.

People Magazine had chosen to feature a beautiful, slightly familiar, blond girl on its cover. I ventured closer to the magazine and saw that she was the sister of a famous supermodel, hence the familiar, but subtly different features. She had died, in her late teens, from asthma. She suffered an attack, and couldn't get to her inhaler on time. I felt like someone had hit me with a taser. Why? I didn't have asthma. I had no family history. But something about this girl, younger than me, who looked so healthy in this picture, really shook me up. Her face haunted me. Even though I had obviously never met her, I couldn't believe she had died, and of something that afflicted half the people I knew.

At lunch, I took the magazine back to the break room. The store frowned on this practice but I felt compelled to know the details. As I read, I learned that people can just develop asthma. It may not necessarily start as a child. I started rubbing my neck. I had been having trouble catching my breath a little lately. It usually happened when my parents argued or felt depressed. The house just felt so heavy, like a thick, dark, hot cloud shrouded us during all regular home activites. Sometimes my breathing felt labored. I thought it was probably stress, but could it be asthma? Didn't stress exacerbate asthma? Maybe stress had triggered the fatal asthma attack with this girl. My nerves kicked in and I lost my appetite. It seemed bizarre that a stranger's life and passing could affect me to such a degree. But it stayed with me for the rest of the day. I tried to avoid eye contact with her image on the magazine but her clear blue eyes peered at me from every check-out stand. I didn't recall People Magazine sitting on every shelf before, yet there she was, looking at me. Her eyes followed me like the dusty, possessed portraits in a haunted house.

After that day, I monitored my breathing. Generally, it's probably safe to say that most of us don't notice our breathing that much. It's instinctual and natural and necessary. I became obsessed. I counted how many times I inhaled and exhaled in a minute, although I wasn't quite sure what the results really indicated. I went into quiet rooms to listen to myself breathe and make sure I heard no wheezing. But I mostly worried about failed attempts to take a deep breath. I would suck in air, and if I couldn't complete the inhalation satisfactorily I would consider it an official episode of inability to catch my breath at all. I would immediately try again. Once I started down that path, it was virtually impossible to relax enough to take a deep solid breath. I would find myself breathing too hard, getting a little light-headed and bordering on hyperventilating. I do not recommend spending a lot of time analyzing your breathing. I was so worried about dying from lack of oxygen, or that I would pass out and nobody would notice to help me, like that poor model's sister, that I forced myself into a spiral of worry and suffering.

I often wonder if the other employees talked about me, discussing why I might be staring at my watch for exactly one minute at a time. I bet they wouldn't guess "breath counting." They probably just thought I eagerly waited for my shift to end. In fact, they likely empathized. We were all clock watchers at various points. I was friendly with everyone, but I wasn't "friends" with any of the other staff. We didn't pick up a burger and see a movie after closing up. But we all smiled at each other, said polite "hello"s, occasionally commented on a customer, and waited for time to hit that magical, scheduled number, when we could take off the polyester and rejoin our normal lives, already in progress.

One man, in particular, always gave off a friendly vibe. He was an older gentleman, probably in his forties, which although not really old, is fairly old for a grocery bagger. Most averaged about fifteen by comparison. But this man came from a Caribbean island, and had an amazingly thick accent. I happen to have an amazingly difficult time understanding any accent. In fact, my husband makes fun of me all the time because I need him to translate any time we go to any other country, or even a local convenience store. I'm terrible and this trait of mine is terrible. I work on it daily. Anyway, I found it impossible to hold a conversation with this man, whose name, by the way, was Dignity. He would always helpfully venture over to my station to bag the customer's groceries, and talk away at me. I would smile and nod. I didn't understand a word. But at least as I focused on trying to figure out his words, I didn't focus on how well I was breathing, and miracle, I could breathe just fine. I continued smiling and nodding at Dignity, not knowing at all what role I played in the conversation. I just politely affirmed his kind sounding words.

The summer came to a close and I loved every minute of my last day. I splurged and bought myself a freshly made deli sandwich and a hot side, as opposed to the Peanut Butter and Jelly that I usually brought, or the banana I bought if I only had a few coins and had forgotten to bring something. A couple of the other employees bought, or found and brought into the break room, a day-old half sheet cake with green flowers and the words "congratulations" scrawled across the top in pink. It looked as if a name had once adorned the cake as well, but had been scraped off and wiped with fresh white icing. As we enjoyed the cake previously intended for someone else, one high school girl, a fellow cashier, asked for my address at college so she could contact me about applying to school and maybe even get more information about Vanderbilt. In all honesty, I felt pretty cool at that point. I would now get to leave and head back to my real world. The others did not get to escape. This was their real world.

*** 

Back at school, in my own little dorm haven, away from the stresses of home, my "asthma" improved. Occupied by the constant flow of activity and general college revelry, I didn't have much time to focus on individual breaths. In fact, I found that I didn't notice very many missed deep breaths at all. I didn't notice any breathing, which meant, Eureka, I was actually doing it correctly. It seemed I might actually learn a lesson here. If I didn't obsess about my mentally conjured problems, they tended not to exist. I would need to try to remember that over and over again. But for now, it seemed to work.

But then in October the asthma returned. One day. Out of the blue. I went to check my mailbox at the student center. As I rifled through my mail, tossing the junk into the trash, I came across an envelope addressed to me in unfamiliar handwriting. No return address. I opened it and found a greeting card, with a black cartoon cat wearing a witch's hat for Halloween. Yay. I love when people remember me during the holidays. Like most college students, I adored getting mail, period. My opinion changed, as I read the inside.

"Dear Cat." First off, who spells my name like that? Was it a joke because of the animal on the card? Hilarious. "I am writing to you to let you know that after all of our good conversations this summer, I would like to be with you and am in love with you. I hope you feel the same way. I have received a raise and now make $7.35 an hour, which will make it easier to support us. I will be making a trip to Nashville with a friend to visit you. Here is my address. I hope to hear from you soon. Love, Dignity."

I stopped in my tracks, covered the card with the other envelopes in my hand so that nobody else would see (not that anyone was even looking) and steadied myself against the wall. I looked around me, like he might already have arrived, waiting along the wall of the student center walkway, with his "friend." When did we have good conversations? I never spoke a word to him. The entire time that I smiled and nodded, he could have been asking me if I liked him "that way," too. I really needed to work on understanding accents. Okay. Let's put this in perspective. So I had a little unwanted attention. What's the big deal? Except, I was completely freaked out by the fact that months had gone by, I suddenly get this card, and he planned to VISIT! That scared me. Left me cold, in fact. Was this what it meant to have a stalker? I immediately put my hand up to my chest. I had a hard time catching my breath. Oh no. I stumbled back to my dorm as fast as my wheezing would allow me so that I could rush to the phone and call my parents. Cell phones hadn't fully taken off yet, so I had to make the journey home first.

My father shared my concerns and barely let me finish my story before he hung up on me to call the grocery store. As I waited for him to call me back, I started thinking. Maybe I had fallen victim to a practical joke. Maybe that high school girl had understood him when he talked to me and thought this would generate a big laugh. Would someone really think that $7.35 would support a couple or a family? It had to be joke. Silly girl. Getting all worked up over a funny little prank. How ridiculous to think that someone would pine silently for a couple of months, then send a goofy card professing love and support. I breathed regularly. That oxygen felt good. Like nature's inhaler. I went out to spend some time with my roommates and try to forget about the episode.

A couple of hours later, my father returned my call.

"Well, that's all taken care of. He won't be bothering you anymore. And it's going into his file in case he tries to do it again to another unsuspecting girl."

"What do you mean? Was that really him who sent the card?"

"Of course it was him. What are you talking about? You're the one who read the card to me. Have you lost your mind?"

"No, I just thought it might have been a joke. Once I started thinking about it."

"Well, it wasn't a joke. He was there when I called the store. The manager confronted him and he confessed the whole thing." Now I felt slightly offended.

"Geez, Dad, it's not like loving me's a crime," I laughed, still a little nervous.

"No, but he's thirty-seven years old. He should not be creeping young girls out like that. He had no right to say he was going to come visit you. Totally unwarranted."

"And how do we know he won't still?"

"I'll make sure they fire his ass." Well, there you have it. "And get this, he was all sad, said that you were always so nice to him and he thought you really liked him. He didn't think he was doing anything out of the ordinary. That was his way of courting you." My dad let out a huge laugh, diffusing his protective anger from mere seconds ago. "Kat, do me a favor and try to know what someone is saying to you before you just nod and agree, 'kay?"

Amazingly, after a month or so, I put the whole Dignity affair out of my mind. For the most part. I can't deny a few times when I would leave campus for something and think that I caught a glimpse of him across the street, watching me. But I managed to keep the "asthma" at bay. I had just enough going on that I forced myself to forget my fear. At least push it down where I couldn't see it. This would be the last time for a long while that I would be able to do that with any success.

Hypochondriac Lesson #9:
Good books and good friends are great diversions.

## 9- Reading Between the Lines

"Look at that torch!" Blaine eyed me coyly as he said the words. "Oh, did that sound gay? Well, so what?!" He started laughing and set the Olympic souvenir back on the shelf.

"You're such a cliché," I said.

"Why, because I'm sassy?"

"That. And your frosted tips and love of Cher."

"She's a Goddess! Don't you dare say anything about my Cher Cher."

"Never," I replied. He seemed satisfied that I wouldn't be insulting his Cher Cher. Today. We would revisit the conversation on many other days.

"Oh, I can't believe that we get to be right here, where all the magic happens," he said wistfully. "The daring feats of physical prowess." He gestured dramatically. "The sob stories of blind mothers and broken bodies. The male gymnasts. Sigh. All in the pursuit of gold. I may cry for two weeks straight."

"Yep, it's pretty cool," I said, as I emptied the box and carefully placed the books and other Olympic inspired objects on the end-cap shelf.

"PRETTY COOL? Have you no heart? No feelings? No American spirit?" He looked like I had crushed his childhood dreams. He knew he wasn't the Olympian, right?

"Oh, I agree. I love the Olympics, too. And it's awesome that they're here in Atlanta, but it's not like I have tickets for anything. I'm going to be watching it all on TV just like I always do. But don't worry," I grabbed his shoulder, encouragingly, "I'll probably have a tear to spare at some point. It never fails. Who can resist the blind mothers?"

"Well, okay then. I was worried. Like your heart might be all black. You seem like a sad little Pussy Kat today."

"My heart is fine, thanks. Full of love, even. And even more so if you'd help me shelve these books." I indicated the three huge boxes of new stock. Mall bookstores, outside of Borders and Barnes and Noble, tended to scale on the small side. I had no idea how we would ever find room for so many new books. But I couldn't complain. Working at this bookstore was like bathing in Nutella. That's a good thing, which you probably already know if you've ever had the taste sensation of this wondrous product. Surrounded by books, a personal love, I could hardly remember the summer days of yore when I worked my heinous other jobs. During slow times, I could venture over to a shelf and discover new authors, new worlds. It was fantastic. Blaine's excitement was perfect, though; the whole Atlanta area buzzed over the upcoming Olympics, which brought everyone together and out of the mundane for at least a little while. Mallrats bonded with Eyeglass Hut employees over the strengths of the American track team. The Chick-fil-A workers got into heated discussions with the girls from Rave over synchronized swimming, and well, Blaine regaled me endlessly with personal facts of the entire men's gymnastics team. These were good times from a community point of view.

At home, not so much. My mother found work at a local hospital doing clerical records work and my father worked in a warehouse, counting inventory in the middle of the night. He had tried to work in the deli of the same grocery store where I had "enjoyed" the previous summer, until he sliced off part of his thumb while cutting some turkey and the managers decided the deed unsanitary and tried to put him on stock. He declined and found alternate arrangements at the warehouse. But with both parents just making hourly wages, and my sister attending daycare, they weren't quite making ends meet and, therefore, not thrilled with life. In my naïve way of thinking, I kind of hoped that the Olympics would lift their spirits. Maybe give them some inspiration. It seemed like all the athletes had stories of times down in the dumps. I wanted my family to take something away from their experiences. Maybe I should've started playing feel good music in the background to get them in the mood to be spiritually lifted.

So far, however, my hope for an Olympic boost had failed. My dad started feeling bad at his job. At first he thought he suffered from fatigue from working through the night. But after a while of his body not feeling quite right, he decided to let a doctor decide.

I had whipped up a batch of Hamburger Helper (I wasn't much of a chef back then) to surprise my parents with dinner one day, when they arrived back from the Doctor's office looking forlorn.

"Kat, I have diabetes."

"Oh."

"They said I need to watch what I eat. And I should try to lose some weight and not be stressed out all the time." He laughed. "Easier said than done, huh?"

"Oh."

"Do you understand what I'm telling you?"

"Well, yeah. But people live with diabetes all the time, right? That's not so bad." I had no idea. I only remembered a girl from my cheerleading squad in the third grade who had it and gave herself shots during each practice. But she seemed otherwise fine. And the doctors had told him before to eat healthier. We'd been through all this already. Like I said, I had no idea.

"You're right. But I do have to be more aware of things now." And we kind of left it at that. Stress levels stayed high, especially when my parents struggled to meet their bills. They didn't exercise. My dad checked his blood sugar periodically, the only indication of change on his part. But he didn't really alter the food on his plate. His reaction seemed about the same as when the doctors handed him the high cholesterol diagnosis. I guess he had no idea, either.

\*\*\*

"Kat, the new Grisham books are in," said my boss. "Let's get those puppies out and get some customers in here. Get Blaine to help you when he gets back from lunch."

"I'm on it." Awesome. I'd been looking forward to the new legal thriller escape. Shoot, I was even thrilled to be working. My parents had fought all morning and when they dropped me off at work (we were down to one ancient car that was paid off), my mother told me she couldn't stand the sight of me as I exited the car. I wasn't even part of the conversation, but I think everything and everyone had turned a culprit in my mother's misery. Not pretty.

I pushed the box over to the display structure with my foot, in an effort to avoid breaking my back at such a young age. For the record, book boxes are extremely heavy; note this whenever you move. I opened up the box and pulled one out, stroking the front and back cover. Oh, how I would love to be an author and get a book published like this. I wanted to inhale it and smell the ink. I placed it lovingly at the top of the display. Perfect. I bent over at the waist and piled a bunch of books into my arms at once and quickly stood up. The room went black. My heart pounded harder and faster than it had at any time in its young history. I grabbed the nearest bookcase so that I wouldn't fall. The dark, midnight curtain over my vision parted slowly, but still left a film, followed by floating spots of watery black. My stomach clenched and without seeing fully, I pushed myself off of the bookcase with my arm and rushed to the back room for employees only. I locked myself in the bathroom and found myself sick for the next twenty minutes. The beat in my chest sputtered and boomeranged and I truly did not believe my body could keep up with it. Once I determined I could leave the back room, I tried to return to the floor to seek help, but I shook violently and took the first chair in my sight.

My boss came to find me, thinking I had opted to extend a break. I guess the new books attracted the lunch crowd and Blaine still hadn't returned. The look on her face as she entered said, "Why are you being so lazy?" When she saw me, though, she stopped and put her hand up to her face in alarm.

"Are you okay?"

"I don't know," I said, grasping onto the seat of the office chair with both hands, as if I might fall right off of it. Maybe I needed a seat belt. I felt the cold sweat on my back and neck, getting chillier as the air conditioning worked to dry my clothes despite my best nervous efforts.

"Call your family. You should go home. You don't look good." That was the understatement of the millennium.

"Okay." The break room spun. My heart continued to hammer away uncontrollably, like a bad rock drum solo that nobody wants to hear; the kind that gives the audience a severe headache, and you find yourself looking at your watch wondering when it might end. Enough already.

I dialed my parents and my mom picked up, sounding more exasperated than usual.

"What!" she snapped into the phone.

"Mom, it's me." I drew a deep breath, still trying to steady myself. I couldn't believe that I was having a heart attack at only twenty years old. I didn't really believe it possible. Yet here I was. My heart. Attacking. I could find no other explanation. The episode lasted too long to mean anything good.

"Uh huh. What do you want?"

"I need you to come get me. I've had some kind of episode and I think I need to see a doctor."

"What's wrong with you?" I told you that I get this question a lot; but this was the first real time. She seemed very annoyed.

"It's my heart. I don't know. I can't get it to calm down. And I was sick. Like stomach sick."

"Well, you probably just ate something that didn't agree with you."

"Can you just come get me? And take me to see someone?" I couldn't believe I had to argue with her. Didn't she hear the fear in my voice? What had happened to my mother?

"Fine. But be outside. I swear, between you and your father…" she trailed off and I heard the phone click as she hung up. As soon as I got past this physical thing I had going on here, I really needed to figure out a way to make my parents happier. Their sadness and anger increasingly took a toll on all of us, coloring our world a very deep and melancholy blue. They needed to do something fun once in a while, like old times.

As I stood outside of the mall entrance with the smokers, trying to avoid inhaling their toxic cancer cloud, supporting my wavering frame up against the wall, as I had no faith that I could stand upright by myself, I felt a second wave of sick approaching. I breathed deeply and ran my tongue over my chapped lips. To distract myself, I grabbed a section of my hair and started braiding. I had to get my mind off my impending death somehow. It didn't work, but it gave me something to do with my hands besides taking my pulse. After what seemed like an eternity, I saw my mom driving in. I could see the frown on her face from the first moment I viewed the car, even at a distance. Her displeasure reached across great distances, vast deserts. I suddenly had a vision of standing on one side of the Grand Canyon, she on the other, and still detecting that look of chagrin and hopelessness. I think she had suffered from a chasm in her very soul, broken and seemingly bottomless. And she had been so happy, so divine, at one point. I could still remember those occasions clearly, so I know it couldn't have been that long ago.

I slid into the car, carefully, slowly. My mother eyed me up and down, and then stepped on the gas to whisk me away to (hopefully) better health.

"I don't like the way you look," she said, her voice softened by many degrees.

"I don't like the way I feel."

"Why don't you tell me exactly what happened." So I did. Then I cried. The tears seemed to spring from nowhere, water from dry earth. A massive surge of release accompanied the deluge and my heart started to calm, its rate on the decline as we continued our conversation, and I wiped the wetness from my stained face with the back of my hand.

"I don't know what's wrong with me, but I've never been so scared in my entire life. I've never felt this way before."

"Well, now's not the best time for any of us to be getting sick. You know?" I shook my head, like I understood, but I didn't. Was there ever a "best time" to get sick? "I guess I sort of thought that with all the other crap that's been happening in our lives, it was okay, because we had our health. But now, with your father...and you," her voice cracked. "Well, you just can't be sick, that's all."

"Okay. I'll try not to be." I tried to laugh a little, but it just sounded like a mucous infested snort. I think fluid came out of my nose for good effect.

\*\*\*

At the doctor's office, the nurse made me strip off my clothes and wrap myself up in one of those shapeless scratchy gowns with designs on them that you never really notice but expect on the fabric; stars or periwinkle flowers. "Open to the front," the nurse indicated which scared me because I didn't have any idea what kind of exam or test they planned to run on me. I felt exposed. Vulnerable.

The nurse knocked on the door after what she presumed a suitable time to change, and entered through the door backward, pulling in a large machine with multiple wires protruding in all directions. Did they plan to electrocute me? Shock me, at least? Read my mind? What in the world? I just hope it's not needles. Please don't be needles.

"What is that?" I asked. My voice actually wobbled, like I had just hit puberty; and was a boy.

"This? This is what we use to do an EKG. Don't worry, it doesn't hurt." She smiled at me, and then her face turned serious. "You look worried. Seriously. Don't be. I'm just going to put a bunch of stickers on you while you lie down. Then the machine will read your heartbeat for a few seconds and that's it. It looks a lot scarier than it actually is. DON'T WORRY!" She looked over at my mother. "Is she always this worried at the doctor's office?"

"Yes," my mother said. But truth told, my mother looked a little worried as well. That didn't abate my fears in the slightest.

"Hmm," replied the nurse. "Well, try to calm down. Things will go a lot smoother if you can relax." Easier said than done, woman. As she started placing the little round electrode stickers, which looked like metal nipples, all over the torso of my corpse-positioned body, I found my thoughts turning to visions of old people in hospital dramas, walking around with plastic wires coming out of their noses, and shuffling down the hall pushing the poll with the medicine bag flowing into IVs. I could now be cast as an extra in "Cocoon." I couldn't have reached that place in my life already. I'm too young to die. I felt woozy and faint.

"Okay, be still."

I held my breath.

"Don't hold your breath. Just breathe normally."

"Oh, sorry." I breathed on command. A few seconds lapsed.

"Alright, that's it. See, not so bad."

"I have to admit, you were right," I said, surprised at my own comfort.

"Now just take a seat and the doctor will be in shortly to go over the results with you and your mom." She wheeled the large machine out again to help it make its journey to read somebody else's heart, a medical fortune teller of sorts.

I sat on the edge of the table and swung my legs back and forth. I looked up at my mother, slightly, so as not to stare directly at her. I felt bad; guilty for making her worry when she already had so much on her mind. She had her eyes cast downward and she absently picked at her nails; defeated. I should just get up, put my clothes back on and tell her false alarm, and let's go home and play a game or something. Maybe go to the ninety-nine cent video store and rent something light and fun. Even if the movie was old, she would still like that. She always enjoyed watching "Bachelor Party." She would laugh until she cried. Something about Tom Hanks and his madcap friends and hints of bestiality tickled my mother's funny bone. I bet they carried that movie.

Just as I opened my mouth to speak, the doctor walked in. She was strikingly pretty, but did she seem a little young?

"Hi there, Kathleen. And you must be Kathleen's mom. I'm Dr. Russo. How are you folks doing today?" We both smiled a smile that said, "Really, do you even have to ask?" She chuckled almost to herself. "Well, I've looked over the EKG and everything looks great. I don't see any problems there. I'm going to take a little listen." She indicated the stethoscope around her neck. "Then we'll get to the bottom of your problem." I followed her instructions for the necessary size of breath. She listened, and then breathed on the little metal disk to make it warmer, when I flinched from the cold shock.

"Does it sound okay?" I asked when she pulled away. This is a common habit I have. When a doctor examines anything, I want to know right away if it's normal.

"Sounds beautiful. With that heart, you'll go another seventy or eighty years." I did the quick math in my head to make sure this sounded satisfactory. Phew! Okay. I was nervous, so give me a break. "Now why don't you tell me exactly what happened. Don't leave anything out." Once I finished, she said, "You had a completely normal response to bending over and picking up stuff. The blood probably rushed to your head, your heart started pumping fast to compensate, and voila, that was that. Now after that initial reaction is where you, and your mind, come in. You panicked. You had what sounds to me like a full on panic attack. Have you been stressed out?"

I looked over at my mom, who turned her head away, then nodded affirmatively to the doctor. She swept her eyes from me to my mom.

"I'm going to prescribe something for you to take so you can try to calm down a little. You don't want to have panic attacks. They're not fun. As you already know. Here, I'm going to give you the first dose now because you still seem really upset." I took the little red pill she offered me and washed it down with water from a mini paper cup. My mother appeared to wince when I swallowed, but I could have imagined that.

"Are panic attacks life threatening?" I had to know.

"Not in themselves. But stress over a long period of time can have long term health effects. Better to address it now."

For the next five days I took the pills. I trudged through work in a fog and fell instantly asleep when I got home. I dozed during TV shows, went back to bed

early and had a hard time waking to my alarm the following morning. Finally, my
parents reached their limit.

"I'm not going to tolerate a comatose daughter walking around," said my
father, angry that I would take "brain pills" to begin with. "You're a little stressed.
So what? So are we and we're not taking anything. You need to stop taking these
crazy pills and start dealing with the real world, girl."

"You can't keep doing this, Kat. You're tired all the time. All you do is
sleep," my mother added. So before the week finished I stopped the pills. And I
definitely woke up again. And I definitely had panic attacks again; every day in
the bookstore for the rest of the summer. I would have dizzy spells, or gasp for
breath. My "asthma" had returned, although it could've been the abundant amount
of dust from the books on the higher shelves; they don't call those dust jackets for
nothing. I grimaced through these episodes and hoped they would pass. If I kept
myself occupied, I could work through most of the day, but I found that I had to
take extra bathroom breaks to splash cold water in my face, or dampen my neck.

"Why do you look so moist?" Blaine asked me.

"Isn't it hot in here?" I would reply.

"Um, not really, Honey. And you might struggle to find a date if you can't get
that sweating thing under control." He moved his hand dismissively up and down
in front of my face.

"I know. I'm working on it." I barely managed to make it through each day.

The real kicker arrived in test form; I had to take the LSATs that summer,
to prepare for Law School applications. While studying, I found that I struggled
with focus because I kept analyzing how hard and fast my heart beat. On the day
of the test, my head felt heavy and I worried I wouldn't have the ability to hold
it up through the whole test. I managed to make it through to the end and score

sufficiently well, even though my mind seemed to work against me. I know I could've done better.

When the Olympics finally arrived that summer, I excitedly watched coverage each night with my family. I thought the diversion would cure me. Instead, I became so involved in the stories of triumph and the outcomes of individual competitions that I would fret about them. I would get physically nervous for the athletes and then worry about having another panic attack. Which would lead to a full blown panic attack. Which would lead to a cold wet towel on my neck and the same across my forehead. Every night. That is just not normal. I kept having these panic attacks because I worried about dying; that I would just pass out, lose my breath, and my heart would stop. I felt on the verge of all of these when I would have an attack. I had created a vicious cycle in my mind. Which came first, the chicken or the egg, the bad feeling or the thought of the bad feeling?

I couldn't wait to get out of this house and get back up to school for my senior year. Something had to give.

Hypochondriac Lesson #10:
Forget about the mountain of worry
and just deal with the individual stones.

## *10- An Almost Affair to Remember*

I was a Lolita. Well not technically. I was of age. But the age difference qualified as a May/December situation. Maybe even April/December. I was the student and he was my professor. I was twenty and by my calculations, because, of course, I would never ask directly, he was late forties; probably around forty-seven. And there was the issue of his pending divorce. Also, technically, we hadn't done anything. So then Kat, you may ask, what are you talking about?

I suddenly found myself thrown into my senior year of college. Where did the time go? Things were just getting good in my second life. This precious haven of a home away from home, especially when "home" didn't feel like the right word for life with my parents, would end in less than nine short months. I faced law school applications and making decisions about the rest of my life. I had no idea where I would go, how I would live; just a blank vast void after graduation. A veritable black hole in a galaxy I couldn't get my head around. Standard stuff for the college senior, but I wanted to bury myself up at the campus pub and devour a whole cheesecake, wallowing in my own uncertainty. I watched as college sweethearts made plans for life after school together. I hadn't found love as I'd originally expected I would in college. I'd discovered a lot about myself, which is good, but I also felt lonely and scared. As you might imagine, my panic attacks followed me around on a daily basis, like a pet, or my soul. My mind cringed and spasmed and longed for soothing. I listened to a lot of Sarah McLachlan during this period.

I took classes that I knew I would love, wanting to savor the last moments of academia; give myself the final opportunity to learn music "From Beethoven to the Beatles" in one semester, for example. I met Him in one of these horizon expanding courses. The Professor. Please try not to get the one from Gilligan's

Island in your head. I thought nothing of him at first. About six feet tall. Graying hair, green eyes, corduroy jackets. He looked pretty typical. On a few of my less lazy days, exercise wise, I'd noticed him in the recreation center using a treadmill, listening to his headphones with his eyes closed. I started to wonder about what went on in his head.

In class, he gave us a project, made us divide into groups and create a product on a current event. We could use whatever setting we wanted and interview anyone. I was thrilled to have something else to do besides sit and take notes three times a week.

My little assigned group of four decided to make a video survey to explore the relationship of the students with the outside community; the community, that is, outside of our little self imposed bubble of college. We wanted to see just how the students connected with the world around them. We found sound bite gold with students during random passerby interviews on campus. We asked how they served or interacted with the community. "I did a walk once…I don't remember for what cause," or "I don't care, I just want to get my parents off my back." These moments tugged at the heart strings and provided faith in mankind. The final video product blew the whistle on student apathy, showcased the gunners of the school, and brought the class to tears of laughter. With a powerful, yet whimsical, overlay of music, I would describe the production as stellar. I think I started to fancy myself a Scorsese, or at least a Ken Burns. And I enjoyed the hours in the editing room working on the piece and the new closeness with the other kids in my group. We met with much praise from the class when the video finished.

A few days later we congregated in Professor's office for the report of his thoughts, both academic and emotional, about our project. He would then bestow our grade upon us. After regaling us with his views on community interaction and reminiscing about the joy of our little documentary, he sighed deeply, making a steeple of his fingers and tapping the steeple against his lips; as if the tapping would bang the right words into his mouth, like Johnny Carson with his envelope.

"I'm going to give you a B-plus." He shuffled some papers on his desk and prepared to stand to show us out the door. "How does that sound?" The other three nodded, silently, in agreement. Now keep in mind, I didn't say an awful lot in class, was rather intimidated by this man, but for some reason, I saw his final question, "How does that sound?", as a challenge; as a door for opportunity. I looked at my fellow group members, slightly appalled at how easily they accepted their fate. Before I even knew that I'd opened my mouth, I spoke.

"Actually, that doesn't sound good at all." Wait, did I just say that out loud? His eyes widened and he stayed in that half up, half down perch, like bending over a doctor's bed waiting for a rectal exam. I don't think he really knew what to do at that point. Finally, he slowly, disbelievingly, sat back down. And yet, even in the uncomfortable silence; although I think one of my group members made an audible gasp; I considered it a fine time to talk more.

"I'm not quite seeing how you can praise every single aspect of our project, consider all the positive evaluation from the class, review the editing room logs, noting that we spent ungodly hours in that tiny room, see that we had perfect sound, perfect lighting (yes, I was on a roll), and perfect flow and still think that it's fair to give us a B-plus." Then I went mute. I cleared my throat. Whew. I needed to get that off my chest. A long pause ensued. My group mates looked like they could have slaughtered me with anything they could dig out of their backpacks, although I'm not sure how their ID cards would have caused much damage. They didn't even have keys to scratch me with. Maybe brain me with a large textbook or something. One fidgeted with her nails, the other looked around the room as if to admire the décor and the boy in my group might have tried whistling nonchalantly. I, however, kept an almost hawkish direct eye contact with Professor. Just when I thought I might soil myself, he did something I did not expect. He crumbled into laughter. The others joined in with nervous, yet overly hardy, laughter as well, through tightened jaws.

"Where did you guys get her?" He looked at me with a "well, I never" kind of look, part amusement, part shock. He had gone almost an entire semester of not knowing me from any other girl in the class. Now he noticed me and everything would change. We talked some more; argued, more accurately. I could feel the imagined hands of the group members wrapping themselves around my neck. I could see it in their eyes when I ventured to look at them.

"Okay, how about an A minus, then." He had caved. I made him CAVE. Nice. Mental high five to myself. As we exited his office, which was significantly warmer by this time than when we had entered, those high fives turned into reality as my group immediately stopped collectively planning my murder and began to sidle up to me like I'd evolved into superstar tough stuff. They congratulated me on turning the events around for the team. I acted all cool.

"He's just a man. With reason. Why should we be afraid of him and think that we can't speak our mind about our grade? We deserved that grade." I didn't add that I might have wet myself just a few drops.

And so the game began. I would go into Professor's office after class to have a good old fashioned disagreement/discussion. I savored my condition of nerves and excitement, the only time I enjoyed my anxiety, before I would enter the room. His face would light up and he would put down whatever he worked on to invite me in; even when he didn't have office hours. At the beginning, I thought nothing of it. I just wanted to keep enjoying the academic discourse. This was the reason

I'd wanted to go to college in the first place; the dream of having passionate and interesting academic conversations with professors. Beer pong had nothing on this. I felt so alive. How considerate of him to so willingly take a student under his wing and mentor so proficiently.

Then one day, I showed up at his office after a school break. I had gotten a haircut and bought a couple of new outfits. I wore one of them on this particular day; a denim skirt and a short sleeve shirt that went to the waist but if I reached for something, would show my midriff; I swear nothing skanky or revealing. I also had my contacts in instead of my glasses, which I usually wore to class. You would have thought I was the mousy, shy girl in the movies who suddenly gets a makeover and lets her hair down out of her pony tail and everyone notices her. I walked into his office and he looked at me differently.

"Wow, Kat. You look…," he trailed off and started going through stuff at his desk. Okay, then. I commenced talking to him about class reading.

"I can see your stomach," he said, paying no attention to the conversation. I looked down and tugged on my shirt, self consciously. "No, it's fine. I've just never seen you…why are you so dressed up?"

"It's just a shirt and a jean skirt. I'm not half as dressed up as the other girls around here. I don't have my pearls on," I said, trying to lighten the mood. He seemed very serious. Every time he looked at me, it felt, well, rather laced with intention. But I had very few skills in the art of seduction, and was, admittedly rather naïve, so even though little red flags waved in my brain and actually developed voices, I ignored them and continued talking. After that day, I kept visiting. I spent hours in that ten-by-ten room, at least three times a week.

When I saw him, I felt less scared about all the other parts of my life. I had started to have panic attacks on a daily basis. Walking to my class, I would experience an out-of-body sensation, where I would think, "Nope, I'm not going to physically make it to class. I'm going to collapse and die right here." My legs lightened, floating or hovering above the ground. My head, shoulders and arms deadened with weight, to the point that I knew I could not hold them up. Dizziness would overtake me. I would gulp huge amounts of air and still not feel like I could get enough oxygen. At restaurants, I would have a hard time looking up because my head felt heavy and I feared my face would hit my plate. I really didn't want noodles in my hair. A friend told me a story of a kid who had stomach pain and died in his sleep of appendicitis. I always had stomach pains and after hearing this story, I would sit up in bed until late at night, rocking like a person in an insane asylum, unable to go to sleep, fearing my own demise in the wee hours of the morning. How long would it take before my roommates found my decaying body? Oh horror. But in Professor's office, I wasn't worried about dying. I spent my time instead deciphering his words, his looks, and his body language. Maybe he saw a strength in me that my body seemed to lack.

One day I meandered down to his office after my last class on a Friday afternoon. Honestly, I'm not even sure why. Just to talk about current events, probably; not even anything related to class. He asked my opinions and seemed to want to hear my replies. I craved more of that attention. Later, as I got ready to leave him, I noticed out of his window that a light rain had started to fall. I commented on it and he immediately jumped up and offered me the coat he'd worn into work that day.

"No, that's okay," I said, feeling the beginnings of something a little funny inside, like a worm slithering around. I guess you could call it butterflies. If butterflies make you want to scream in ecstasy and race to the bathroom with diarrhea at the same time.

"Please, I insist. I don't want you getting wet. Or worse." He walked around his desk and behind me to hold it while I slipped my arms into the sleeves. Oh my god. This is some weird version of the boyfriend jacket. The coat hung on my frame loosely. Frankly, I swam in it, and people would know that it clearly did not belong to me.

"But how will I give it back to you? Won't you need it?"

"It doesn't matter. I'm sure you'll find some way to get it back to me." I felt a jolt travel all the way through my body and stop to radiate in my lower abdomen; tickling little spiders in my nether regions.

As I walked back to my dorm I hugged the coat around me. It smelled of age and distinction, musk and academia, and a hint of high quality cologne, all in an aggressively appealing way. As I walked into my suite (I lived with five other girls in a dorm suite), a look of suspicion crossed my roommate, Marianne's, face.

"What is that you're wearing there?" She asked with a nod of her chin in my direction.

"It appears to be a coat," I said.

"Uh huh. And who does that coat belong to?"

"Well I was having a class discussion with Professor and he suggested I take it since I didn't have a raincoat." I don't know why I felt the need to specify it as a class discussion. Or rather, why I felt like I needed to LIE about it being a class discussion. It didn't matter. Marianne had a general mistrust of the whole situation anyway.

"You know that's not really appropriate."

"What, wearing a raincoat?"

"Him…lending you his raincoat."

"He was just being nice to a student. He would've done the same for any student in his office today. I just happened to be the one there."

"Sure, you keep feeding yourself that BS." And off she went to another room, although as she walked away, I distinctly heard her say something to the effect of no other student having the chance to be there, since I was always there. She really excelled at mumbling, so I can't be sure. I could've been projecting. Saturday morning, however, I returned from breakfast to find my bed made (an unusual occurrence) and sexual harassment pamphlets printed by the University meticulously fanned across the comforter.

***

I should have stopped talking to him. But it's not like I considered myself any sort of temptress. As fate would have it, Professor just so happened to teach an extremely interesting class the following semester that I felt compelled to take. He began the class by designating me the leader of the class project, a position that would require me to keep tabs on all of my classmates' work progress. They would have to report to me, and I would inevitably hold the sole responsibility for the project's integrity. So why did he choose me?

"You have to understand," he said to the class. And was that a lascivious smile in my direction? "I have a special relationship with Kat." Then he moved on to something else, while I sat in red, heated, humiliated silence, the rest of the class casting glances in my direction. I could already see them whisper the words, "sleeping together." Oh right hell. What had I gotten myself into? I went home that day with a headache of Superman proportions. My stomach burbled and the room rotated. A normal person would have instantly had the common sense to know that these symptoms stemmed from the nasty stress instigator in my head. But my "special relationship" was such a new experience for me that I didn't have the clarity of thought to see the connection.

The following week, Professor held class in a computer lab to teach us about a program that would aid us in our project. When I had a question, he came over to me, rested his hands on my shoulders, leaned down so that his chest brushed gently and tantalizingly against my back and his head hovered right next to mine. When he spoke his answer, he did so softly and directly into my ear. I felt the hairs stand up on my neck and electric fingers venture up and down my spine. I could almost sense the five o'clock shadow on his usually smooth face trying to connect with my cheek, like a cat's whiskers sensing any foreign object nearby. My pupils dilated felinely. And darn it, there went my heart again. Bump, bump bump, bump. Now three times fast in a row, before steady rhythm. My head conducted an inner fencing spar, where the blades threatened to protrude from my eyes. Before standing all the way back up, his hands warmly and subtly massaged my shoulders; a fleeting millisecond he thought the others couldn't see. Who was he kidding? This was juicy. I would be interested to know if my professor was sleeping with a student and so were they. I had zero friends in that class. Nobody wanted to talk to me. And I couldn't blame them. He made it so obvious. Except, wait! We WEREN'T sleeping together.

Our first exam came and went, and I found myself staring at a bluebook with a large "B" circled in red pen on the front cover. Annoyed, as I had really studied for this exam, I flipped through the pages and found little to no comment or correction. After class I hastened to his office, with attitude at the ready. That was how he liked it, remember?

"What is the meaning of this?" I asked, suddenly sounding a little like Sigourney Weaver in "Working Girl." I was tough and in charge. I threw the bluebook down on his desk for effect. He took the bait. I could see the hint of a smile. This was what he had wanted, expected.

"What do you mean?" Okay, I'll play along.

"Why did I get a B? You had nothing bad to say about my answers. I know I was thorough. So why didn't I get an A?" I crossed my arms and pursed my lips. I was taking no crap. He grabbed my bluebook, theatrically, as if forcing himself to take another look against his better judgment. He sat back in his chair for a quick read through, and then cautiously returned the exam to his desk.

"If I gave you an A, I thought it would look bad to the rest of the class."

"What the HELL?" I said. Then I quickly covered my mouth. I never used cuss words in front of adults. I understand that I was twenty at the time, and technically an adult myself. But for some reason, I still never used foul language in front of people older than me, and absolutely not once in my life in front of my parents; which is funny, really, because my father swore like a sailor, up and down, right and left. All the time. If he could find thirteen ways to say something, he would choose the way with the most offensive words. I used to make him pay me for saying bad words. I developed quite a collection of coins for a while; until he got angry when I called him on it, and held my hand out waiting for payment. He vehemently exclaimed, quite cussingly, that he would no longer pay me for his verbal dalliances. Professor appeared taken aback by my potty mouth at this juncture. I could tell by his look. He wanted to scold me like a daughter.

"Why would it matter what grade you give me?" I asked, in a much calmer tone.

"I just thought it would look suspicious. The class already thinks we have a special relationship. I didn't want them to take that further in their minds."

"Oh my GOD. The only reason they think that is because YOU TOLD THEM THAT!" My breath came more heavily now. I thought I might pass out. "YOU said we had a 'special relationship' and now they all think we're sleeping together. That is not MY fault. I should get the grade I deserve. Which is an A. And by the way. It is MY grade. Nobody will ever know what I get. Unless you plan to tell them that, too." I sat down in a huff. I had been standing, and pointing and gesturing, this whole time and I suddenly desired to sit more than anything else in the world. Professor sat quietly for some time.

"Kat, if you want the A, I'll give you the A. I would do anything you asked me to do." I sat, stunned, chilled, heated, sick, elated. I had no idea how to respond. None. For once in my life, and especially in this most unique, nay, special, relationship, I could find no words to say.

"I know they all think we're sleeping together," he continued. "But I leave that as up to you. I will do what you want." He looked a little pale and ill himself. Wait, did he just proposition me? Did he really just say that it was up to me whether we would start ACTUALLY sleeping together? I did the only thing I could think of. I pretended I hadn't heard him.

"Thank you for seeing things my way, and thank you for changing my grade," I said. He looked slightly taken aback, but said nothing further. I left.

On my way home to my dorm, I had to sit down on the grass, for fear of vomiting my last three meals. My head ached so badly, that I knew I must have the dreaded brain tumor I had always feared. It had been, what, about three weeks of this headache? I couldn't believe that I'd just ignored his words. Coward. Would I really want, or be capable of having this secret fling with Professor? Of course, would it be a secret if everyone already suspected it, including my roommates? "What do you do in his office for three hours?" I was enamored, enchanted and completely flattered that a professor found me attractive. A fantasy. Van Halen wrote songs about being hot for teacher. Movies showed the seduction of the young ingénue and the worldly older professor. It felt too easy, a cliché. But the other truth was that I remained a virgin. That's right, I still had not completed the deed. How awful to lose it to a more-than-middle-aged married man with a power position over you. I clearly couldn't head down that road. It didn't help that I had run into his wife once at his office. Shook her hand. Introduced myself. No. I simply could not go there. And I knew he couldn't either.

As I sat on the grass, I put my head between my legs to quell the dizziness. This was it. I would keel over and die all because of adulterous thoughts. Oh the shame. My parents would be so disappointed. My father would not understand.

I stood up, changed direction and walked straight to Student Health.

"I think I have a brain tumor," I cried, with actual tears, when the doctor came into the room. He "there, there'd" me and told me to sit on the edge of the bed while he looked into my glistening eyes and listened to my irrational rationale. He made me stand and hold my hands out in front of me and close my eyes. He instructed me to stretch them out to the sides. He directed me to walk a straight line across the floor. Does he think I'm drunk? Is he going to administer a breathalyzer next?

"Listen," he said, in his best reassuring voice. "I can tell you right now. You don't have a brain tumor."

"But how can you be sure?" I asked.

"You don't have any of the symptoms. I understand that you've been having headaches, but you would be having other problems as well if it was a brain tumor. And by the things you've been telling me and the symptoms you've been experiencing, my best suggestion is to maybe make an appointment with the counselors on campus. I think it would really help you with your stress levels." Quack!

But I listened to him and made my appointment. During my first visit, the counselor told me that I not only had anxiety and more than my fair share of hypochondria, but that I was "textbook" for both.

"So it's 'textbook' to have stomach aches so bad that you can only eat plain baked potatoes, or plain cans of corn?" Yes, I had taken to opening a can of corn or green beans for dinner, no spice, just drained and microwaved. I just couldn't take the stomach burn anymore.

"Your picture could be right next to the definition entries in this book right here," she said, gesturing to a medical tome in her lap. She pointed to an open page that discussed panic attacks. She was a little too chipper for my taste. She gave me a small card to keep in my wallet that outlined what I needed to do when I had an episode. Oddly, one of the entries was not "Dial 911." She must have accidentally left that out.

Hypochondriac Lesson #11:
Sometimes the worst can happen
but it doesn't mean that you're next.

*11- The Night the Lights Went Out in Florida*

This is the part I've been dreading. This is the part I don't like to talk about. This is the part where all of my fears and worries about death turned into a most horrible reality. This is the part when my mother dies. I would rather eat lead paint chips or poke myself in the eyes with a pointed backscratcher than ever live through this sort of thing again. I share it with you so that you will understand how this can affect someone with my particular idiosyncrasies. I also share it with you because I miss her, this amazing woman. Her death altered my life forever, for better or worse.

    \*\*\*

"Breathe, Mom, breathe!" I leaned my head over my mother's prone body, hoping to hear some sign of life. Hearing nothing, I put my lips to hers and blew five quick breaths. Then I placed my shaking hands on her sternum and started to compress, hoping more than anything that I remembered the right way to resuscitate. I had taken CPR in Health class in high school. I'm not sure I paid proper attention; too embarrassed about kneeling on the floor over the dummy in my mini skirt in front of the class. I wish now that I hadn't been as concerned about showing my rear end. Seems unimportant in hindsight.

Oh my God, when are they going to get here? Didn't I call 911 five hours ago?

At three in the morning, I had woken up, startled. My father stood over me, shaking my shoulders, and in a hysterical voice I'd never heard before told me to get up quickly, that something was wrong with my mother. I ran into my parents' bedroom to see my mother standing at a tall chest of drawers, holding on to the edges, her breathing erratic and raspy. It didn't sound like she could catch her breath at all.

"Mom, are you okay?" I had asked, trying to control the frantic undertones, and not succeeding.

No answer, just a piercing look directly back at me, but seemingly without comprehension of who actually stood in front of her; like a zombie. I noticed that she was playing with her wedding ring, absently sliding it on and off, over and over. She could have been standing in line at the bank, bored. She finally slid it off for good and set it on top of the chest. So we'd know where to find it? My father had gone into the kitchen to get some water for her and I could hear him talking to her, asking if maybe she thought it could be asthma or something like that.

"People can suddenly get asthma, Joanie. Maybe that's all it is." I could tell he didn't believe his own words. And in my extensive research of asthma, this didn't seem to fit the bill.

She turned her head towards me. One last look. Suddenly, her eyes rolled back in her head, a silent slot machine, and she slumped into me, like a police protester, as I stood right in front of the bed. I couldn't handle the weight. I felt myself falling and knew she would land on top of me. The term "dead weight" started to make sense to me. The heaviness overpowered my muscles and my breath.

"DAD," I yelled. "DAD PLEASE HURRY, I THINK SHE'S PASSED OUT!"

My father came running in and grabbed his wife and tried to sit her down on the bed. He maneuvered her up against his side as she had gone completely limp.

"Should I call 911?" I asked, terrified. I had never done that before. Were there rules? I didn't want to cry wolf, or get in trouble for putting anyone out.

"I don't know, but I think so. I just don't know what's going on," he said in a panicked, thick voice. "Please Joan, wake up baby, wake up." He rocked her back and forth, gently patting the side of her face. Isn't that what they do in the movies, lightly slap the victim's face until they come to?

I ran into the front room, to the phone and dialed the number, willing the operator to pick up as quickly as possible. Come on, come on, come on. PICK UP THE DAMN PHONE! Finally someone answered. A woman with an infuriatingly calm and slow voice.

"I need someone to come right away," I said, practically screaming.

"Calm down and tell me what's happened," said the woman.

"Please, my mother is unconscious. She was breathing weird, then her eyes rolled…" I couldn't finish as the cry restricted my speech, tightening around my throat like a boa constrictor. I could only see her blue eyes, disappearing. It's still one of the most vivid memories in my mind, so many years later. A photograph on the internal message board of my brain. I will never lose that image.

"Give me the address and we'll dispatch someone right away." Finally.

I obeyed and gave the information, then slammed down the phone, angry at the operator's relaxed demeanor. Couldn't the stupid woman tell there was a crisis here? When I hung up I ran to the front door to open it so that the paramedics would have easy access. I wanted to eliminate any confusion as to which duplex needed the help. The towering thunderheads that so often formed in the Central Florida summertime had been building menacingly that evening. As if sensing my mother struggling for life, they suddenly released large, violent drops of hail and rain. Thunder and lightning crackled fiercely through the early morning sky, lighting up the otherwise silent and peaceful neighborhood street.

I dashed back into the bedroom again to see if my father had made any progress, but he had only succeeded in laying her down on the ground.

"I think we need to do CPR, but I don't know how," he said, crying.

"I can try, but it's been so long since I learned it. I've never had to do it on anybody before."

"It's our only hope until the medics get here. I don't understand what's going on." Neither did I.

So that's how I found myself bent over my own mother, willing the life to return. I kept alternating between using my mouth and my hands, just as they had shown us in the demonstration and practice. I had to repeatedly wipe the wetness from her face where my own tears had dropped down onto her skin. Finally, after hearing what must have been a rib cracking, I guess my father couldn't watch the fruitless effort anymore and pulled me off of her.

"Just go out in the living room and watch for the ambulance. It's not working in here." His choked voice felt like a punch to my stomach. I moved towards the door and stood there staring out, swaying back and forth, unsure what to do with my own body, feeling the exhaustion in my arms. It's amazing how much strength it takes to attempt resuscitation.

Too afraid to enter the room again with my mother and father, I grabbed my rain jacket and braved the elements outside to make sure the ambulance knew where to stop and wouldn't pass up the house. Looking at my watch compulsively, I saw that barely three minutes had passed, although it felt more like thirty. The rain beat down on the plastic hood of my coat, like the sound of a million little bb's and I tried to take shelter under the duplex neighbor's carport closer to the road. Moments later flashing lights from the ambulance emerged from around the corner and I waved my arms back and forth to get their attention. I felt like an unlucky film extra in the middle of the night trying to hitchhike in some horror movie, where the audience is screaming at me for my stupidity at occupying the wrong place at the wrong time. I think I would've preferred that situation to my current one. Two men jumped out of the truck as it stopped in the street and walked toward the house. I screamed at them over the weather to run, please, my mom lay dying. When I re-entered the house, my six-year-old sister, Katrina, stood in the doorway of her room wide-eyed, yet still sleepy. "Sissy, what's happening?" was all she was able to say with her small voice. I quickly grabbed her to shield her from the scene about to take place.

The rest of the night drifted in and out, like I was only conscious part of the time. Later I would recall that more paramedics appeared at the front door to help, but not how many in total. They moved my mother out of the bedroom and laid her in the middle of the living room floor, their temporary emergency tableau. They cut her night gown off for ease of access to her body for resuscitation. Pacing in and out of the room, as I couldn't stomach standing in one place for any length of time, I vaguely remembered seeing electric paddles on my mother's bare chest and hearing medical terms that I didn't understand. Finally, they brought in a stretcher and put her in the ambulance to take her to the hospital. It took four men to lift and carry her. They reminded me of pallbearers. My father followed them out the door and told me to stay put. I had no idea why he asked me to stay, but I didn't question the order and just sat down instead, suddenly deflated. I felt as if some invisible force had ripped out part of my body, my insides exposed, shredded and ready for parasites to devour, but shock had not quite allowed me to feel the pain. Just ravaged and hollow. An emotional corpse.

The young EMT who remained to clean up the rest of the medical supplies called in the situation to somebody that I could not guess. Was there a main 911 depot, where they reported their findings? Speaking into his walkie-talkie, he said, "I'm getting ready to leave the site, with one expired." He stopped abruptly and glanced over at me, holding a confused and scared child in my arms, realizing what he'd just said. "Look," he said, "I don't, um, know that for certain, but they just require me to call in the situation." I just continued to stare at him, not even really digesting anything he said. "I'm sorry," he blurted, and then paused, "but I can't stay here any longer. Are you okay by yourself? I'm really sorry."

I'm not sure if I responded to him or just continued with a fixed expression. The EMT left without another word and I stayed stationary for some period of time. My family had only arrived at this place, the house of Dad's old friend, Mickey, three days before, after deciding they didn't want to stay in Atlanta. They had missed Florida and thought they could try again, maybe in another suburb of Orlando. Our stay was to last temporarily with this nice single man, until my parents could piece their lives back together and get jobs. They had lost the business, lost their house, and according to my mother, their dignity. Mickey had one bedroom, my parents occupied the other, my sister and I slept on the fold-out couch. We all shared one bathroom, a dinette table and a single carport.

My mom and I had stayed up quietly in the small duplex that night to watch Letterman and see a popular guest. I now wish I'd paid more attention to the moment of shared laughter with my mom. But I can't even remember the guest. I do know we had laughed and chatted throughout the broadcast. Then when she noticed me yawning through drooping eyelids, she had said her goodnight. My sister was already snoring. I could never have known that saying goodnight to my mother at that point would be the last opportunity I would have.

As Katrina and I sat in the suddenly empty, dark space, an hour or more may have passed in silence, broken only by the girl's worried sniffling. The noise of my father busting into the door finally jolted me out of my daze.

"She's gone," he wailed, tripping over the furniture and trying to remain steady on his feet, while clutching at his mouth with one hand to control the crying that began to gurgle in his throat. "Oh my god, she's gone. What happened?

How did this happen?"

I did not move; frozen into instant sculpture. Instead, my dad stumbled towards me and crumpled down to the floor next to my chair and grabbed at my arms and legs, anything he could hold onto, however clumsily, and started to weep. I looked up and noticed for the first time that Mickey silently stood behind my father, having followed him slowly in from the car. Tears dripped down his face.

"What do we do now?" My dad asked us.

I uttered my first words since the paramedics first arrived. "I don't know, Dad. I have no idea." I swallowed hard, tasting bile.

My sister reached out with her little hands to embrace her father. "It's going to be okay Daddy. I promise."

***

After the sun came up a few hours later, I found myself sitting in a silent living room with Dad and Mickey, hearing the rest of the world begin its day, oblivious to what had happened the night before. We could hear car doors shut and engines turn over as neighbors headed out to work. Fatigue had finally overcome my sister an hour before and she lay sprawled out on her stomach on the floor at my dad's feet. I wished she would lay somewhere else as I could hardly stomach seeing someone else I loved on the floor, but I knew the girl needed some peace. I looked up at the mask of my dad's face and finally braved the question that I had feared asking the most.

"Um," I said, voice cracking from built up tears, "how...how did it happen? What was wrong with her?" I aimed the questions at nobody in particular. I had a hard time grasping that I now needed to talk about my mother in the past tense.

"Well," Mickey said, nervously clearing his throat, "the doctors said she had congestive heart failure. Her lungs filled with fluid and..." he trailed off, unable to speak, his face crumpling.

"So her back pain?" I inquired in a tremulous voice.

Mickey nodded his head and said in a low, solemn voice, "Yeah, that was part of it. They said she'd probably been having tiny heart attacks for weeks."

"Ah," I breathed, fresh tears springing to my eyes. How could we have missed this? My mother had suffered so extensively right under our noses and we had failed to see the real problem. But then, when I really thought about it, hadn't the signs been there all along and we just didn't understand them? Hindsight is twenty-twenty, isn't that the saying?

I thought back to the previous month when my parents had picked me up at the airport at the end of school. My mother had appeared pale and withdrawn when she used to always have a smile on her face and an upbeat disposition. She had made no effort to style her short wavy hair, with more visible grays than necessary for a woman in her early forties, and she wore loose fitting clothes that she might wear to clean the house.

"Oh god." My mother had audibly winced as she tried to settle into the front seat of the car in the airport parking garage.

"What's wrong mom?" I had asked. "Are you okay?"

"I think I pulled something in my back." She breathed shallowly. "It's been keeping me up at night for a couple of weeks."

"Have you been to see a doctor? It really looks like you're uncomfortable," I had said.

"Nah, it's probably just a muscle thing. I'm going to see a chiropractor next week. That'll fix me right up." She had fidgeted in her seat, trying to attain a more comfortable position, then settled for slumping forward so that no part of her back touched the cushion. I had watched, curiously, as she made an effort to throw her right arm over her left shoulder and push at various spots on her back in an attempt to locate the pain source. Her breathing had seemed labored.

On the day we had loaded the truck to move down south and in with Mickey, my mom had made her trip to the chiropractor to pursue some pain relief. About an hour after her appointment time the chiropractor's office had called and asked my dad to come pick her up, as she was in no shape to drive herself. Concerned, we had rushed over to the office just as an assistant escorted her out of the front double doors. As I looked at my mother, I thought I had never seen a person look so gray and ashen. I felt frightened and shaken at the sight. My mom stared right through us, disoriented, almost as if she didn't recognize us. I swallowed nervously and looked over at my father. He didn't return my gaze as he quickly hurried over to aid my mom.

As he guided her into the car by her arm, the assistant motioned for me to come talk to her in private.

"Listen, is that your mother?" she had asked, nodding her head towards the struggling woman.

"Yes," I replied looking around towards the car.

"Well you need to get her to a doctor. You should do it as soon as possible." She gave me a stern, meaningful look. But there was sadness behind it. "I don't know what's wrong with her, but it's not her back. And she's in some serious pain."

"Okay," I had said, noticing how hoarse I suddenly sounded. "Thank you for your help." Dazedly, I headed towards my parents.

When I got into the car, I relayed this message of advice to both of them. But my mother just weakly shook her head in denial.

"I'll be fine," she had said. "Once we get situated and get some insurance lined up from a full-time job, I'll go to the doctor right away. I promise. But we're literally moving, again, tomorrow and there just isn't a chance for me to go see anyone right now. Besides, we'll need all our money right now for other things." She winced and sucked in a breath, clearly uncomfortable. But I had said no more. Stupid, stupid, stupid. My mother had her mind made up and we had sat in silence for the rest of the drive back to the house. She died three days later.

\*\*\*

Now I looked at my father through red burning eyes.

"So, how could she have been having heart attacks and not known that she needed to go to the doctor? I just don't understand. None of this makes sense to me."

He wiped his eyes and tried to regain composure as he spoke, but his words tumbled out as a choked sob. "She did go to the doctor two months ago. While you were still in school." He struggled to continue, not looking at me and my shocked expression. "They heard an irregularity in her heart, but they said it could be caused by the extreme pain she was in. They told her she should come back in for a stress test, but she just never made the appointment. She felt like we didn't have the money for more doctors' bills and she didn't want to take the time off of work to go in and run on a treadmill. She said she already knew she couldn't run on a treadmill so what more would they be able to tell her? I think she really believed it was just very bad back pain." He hunched over with his head in both hands and tried to stifle the brewing tide.

"I can't believe this," I said, heaving. Oh my God! She went to the doctor, they found the problem, and she STILL died? All previous panic attacks and fears of death were all just a precursor to now. I couldn't breathe. COULD NOT BREATHE!

"We didn't think it was serious. And you know how stubborn your mom is," he said, catching himself, "was. Oh God, do you think I would've let it go on like this if I'd known? What am I supposed to do now? How am I supposed to go on without your mother? She's everything to me. Was…everything."

I bit my lip and turned my head. I couldn't look at him. "I don't know. I'm not even sure what we're supposed to do right now. We've got to tell Grandma and the family, but there's no way I can do it. I mean, I feel like I'm going to throw up."

"Mickey said he would help." I looked over at Mickey and he nodded mournfully. "He's going to help me make the, um, arrangements. Your mother and I never made plans for this kind of thing and we don't really have the money for a burial, so she'll be cremated and we can have her ashes scattered at sea. She always liked the ocean, right?" He didn't wait for me to respond. "You can come with us to the funeral home tomorrow."

"I don't think so," I said, shaking my head rapidly side to side, like a stubborn child who doesn't want a bath or to go to bed. "I don't think I can handle that. If it's all the same to you, I'll stay here with Katrina."

My dad furrowed his brow, clearly crushed, but slowly nodded his acceptance. I didn't think I could physically enter a place where they burned the bodies of loved ones. To me, it all seemed so medieval and left me with a horrible disgust that permeated my whole body. I imagined men dressed in black, masks and everything, throwing bodies into the fire and watching them burn. No thanks. I'd rather pretend something else, anything else, was going to happen than that reality.

Mickey and my father made all the calls to relatives and friends that they could. My dad broke down with each call as if telling the news for the first time. "Something terrible has happened and Joan is gone." But he progressively sounded more defeated with each call. I didn't eat that day, or the two days after, except a couple of saltines, even when Mickey would specifically buy bland food for me.

Death can put you on quite a diet. Visitors started to pour in, people I had not seen or spoken to in ages, to pay their respects and make sure that we could handle our grief. That would be a resounding NO. I seldom spoke. The visitors tried to fill the obvious void with stories of my mother to illustrate their fondness for her and remind me of how wonderful she was. But it felt too soon. I hadn't even begun to accept that my mother would never return. In my mind, she could have simply taken a short trip somewhere. One of her beloved cruises, maybe.

Once all guests finally departed on that first evening, I laid down in the bed. My eyes could barely close, through their painful, swollen lids. They felt sunburned and full of sand. Each time I tried to sleep, my mind flashed back to the horror of my mother lying in the middle of the floor with the EMTs hovering over her. I couldn't seem to quiet the images and noises that replayed in my mind. I kept visualizing how I had pulled my sister into the laundry room to obstruct her view and keep her innocent eyes from witnessing the horror of the EMTs stripping away my mom's nightgown with large shears to get to her bare skin. So barbaric. Almost pornographic. After some time I must have finally dozed off because I opened my eyes with a start to find daylight seeping in through the cheap cream-colored blinds of Mickey's guest room. I sat up slowly, my body still shackled with the weight of sleep, but feeling as if I hadn't slept at all. Legs thrown over the side, I pushed myself out of the bed and shambled down the hall towards the kitchen. My dad sat at the breakfast table staring at a newspaper, but obviously not reading any of it. He likely could not have told me the headline on the front page.

"Kat, I really need you to come with me today. I don't think I can go by myself. I know Mickey will be there, but you're my daughter, her daughter, and I just need you to help me make the decisions for everything. Mickey's neighbor will watch Katrina so she'll be alright. Okay?" He looked up at me, almost pleading.

I cleared my throat. I don't think I can, I wanted to say. I gently pulled out one of the rolling dinette chairs at the table and sat down on the vinyl cushion, running a nail across fake wood veneer. I glanced at my father who, at the moment, embodied helplessness and devastation. I recognized that look, cavernous, depleted, from the one in my own eyes I'd seen in the bathroom mirror the night before. I could not abandon my father at this point, even though a visit to the funeral home was the absolute last thing I thought I could face. Didn't he know who I was? Didn't he understand that I couldn't DO these sorts of things? I couldn't handle illness and death. But he now had nobody else but me. We needed to be there for each other.

I reluctantly nodded my head. "Okay, I'll go." I didn't say anything else, but rose from the chair and walked back to the bedroom to attempt to make myself presentable. No small feat.

\*\*\*

The funeral home offered a more welcoming reception area than I had expected. I had never been inside of one of these places before. Both of my grandfathers had died when I was only a small child and up until now, fortune had blessed the family with no deaths of friends or relatives. I didn't deal well with hospitals where everyone lay sick, for obvious reasons, and I fully anticipated not faring any better in a place where everyone lay dead. Inappropriate in this particular situation, I couldn't stop imagining myself in a coffin. Then my mind took me to side-by-side coffins with my mother. Then I remembered the cremation, and I only felt distress.

A funeral director stepped out of an office upon our arrival and greeted us warmly. He shook my hand, covering the clasp with his other hand and said, "I'm so very sorry for your loss." I mumbled a small "thank you" in return, and followed him, along with my father and Mickey, into a private room to discuss details for my mother's eternal rest.

The director, Robert, gestured to a table with a cluster of chairs and we all took a seat. I scanned my eyes around the room. Soothing, bland, landscape paintings with muted colors adorned the walls, small Grecian columns occupied the corners, and several bright flower arrangements were scattered around the room, all presumably in an effort to infuse the proper amount of respectful cheer, given the subject matter. I focused back on Robert, with his startling black hair framing a face that indicated a man obviously in his late fifties. He must have colored his hair. He looked almost unnatural. But I supposed that given the unnatural appearances of the other occupants of the building, Robert's was not out of place. I started to bounce my knee up and down, anxiously, and chew the skin on each side of my fingernails, going through the line of fingers methodically, like eating corn on the cob. First the left hand, then the right hand. I hope I hadn't caught any germs from this place before sticking my hands in my mouth. Who knew what all the patrons had died from? But if dead, could they still transmit germs?

"David, Kat, I know this is a very difficult time," Robert said with practiced sincerity. "I'm here to try to make your decisions as easy as possible. I know you've stated that you would like for there to be a cremation, so I need you to sign some papers to that effect and you'll need to choose one of the available vessels to hold the ashes."

"We'd like to arrange for the ashes to be scattered at sea," whispered my dad.

"Very well, then let me get your signature here." Robert handed my dad a pen and pointed to a designated line on the form. "And now you have the chance to view the body which arrived early this morning. She's already been made up so that you can see her. But we tell everyone this, and we feel we must tell you the same; she will not look exactly like you remember her. You'll know it's her, but I just don't want you to be startled by the change in her appearance. We had to add extra makeup to cover up the bruising from the masks that they used when they tried to help her."

I felt the bile rising into my throat and knew I wouldn't be able to hold it down. I quickly pushed back my chair. "I'm sorry, I can't be here," I said, and rapidly left the room. I shoved through the front double doors and ran toward a grassy area that overlooked a small pond. I fell to my knees, retching and heaving. Nothing came up, but I couldn't stop the gagging. Out of nowhere the sobs poured out of me. A train of sobs, previously undetected in the tunnel of my body, but which now came roaring to life, enough to wake the neighboring villages. I couldn't see and could barely breathe. Tremors radiated through my limbs that seemed to penetrate to my core. I rested my arms and forehead in the grass, finally giving in to the torrent of emotion. A minute later I heard the doors open and footsteps running towards me, softening as they went from the sidewalk to the grass. Mickey rushed to my side and dropped down to one knee, draping an arm across my back to try to comfort me.

"Kat, are you all right? What am I saying? Of course you're not. Oh boy. This is just so awful. Please Kat, try to get up. Can you do that? Look at me." He gently put his hands on both of my shoulders and pulled me to face him. "Kat, I know it doesn't seem like it right now, but I promise you, everything's going to be okay. You just have to get through the next few days and then you can take some time for yourself to try to get through your grief. I'm here for you and I'm here for your dad," he said encouragingly.

"Mickey, I can't go look at her. I just can't. It's not her. It's just a shell and I

don't think I can look at that with whatever artificial makeup they've put on her."
I gulped for air, wishing for a brown paper bag to help me stabilize. "She couldn't
swim," I cried. "Her ashes are going out to sea and she couldn't even swim." My
body continued to involuntarily convulse.

"It's okay. Just breathe. Just breathe. Listen, you don't have to go back in
there. But I think your dad wants to see her, so you may be out here for a little bit.
But it's okay, you don't have to go in there if you don't want to," he said.

I nodded and looked up at Mickey, this dear man, as he tried to wipe some of
the tears away from my face, attempting to keep me stable by holding on to me. I
finally told him that I would be fine, and to go back inside since I was sure that my
father would need him. "I'm sorry Mickey," I said suddenly. "I'm sorry this had to
happen to you, in your house. You don't deserve to be put through this. You're a
good friend. Thank you." He stood up, gave me a tentative smile and walked back
inside.

I managed to perch myself upright against the thick trunk of a shady willow
tree in the front lawn of the funeral home. I stared in a trance, watching the
lively Orlando traffic zoom by in such direct contrast to the stillness inside the
funeral home. I remained stationary out there while my dad finished making the
arrangements and went to view my mother's body. I tried to suppress my nausea
as I thought of him bent over his wife, crying quietly over her placid, waxy face.
Would it even look like her? Would it give him the illusion that she's just sleeping?
I reflected sorrowfully on the fact that my final image of my mother would always
be that of a near-lifeless, half-nude body carried out on a stretcher.

\*\*\*

Two days later, we held the funeral for Joan Marlow Dawson. I did not expect
the seventy-plus people who turned out for the event. I had forced myself to stand

at the entrance door to greet the guests and was startled by the long-lost friends and distant family members who arrived to pay their respects. Not too long ago my family had been well known and important in the local community, but the failed business and a bankruptcy had changed all of that. When the terrible reality of the situation finally had hit my parents, they had to vacate their home and give up one of their cars.

I recalled the day the men came to repossess the car. My mom shut herself in the master bedroom that was no longer hers and cried.

"Don't cry, Joanie, baby," my dad said through the door. "I'm going to make this right. You'll see." But things had not improved and our family had disengaged from everyone they knew in the community. To see these people from our past in this venue was just plain strange.

I did not shed any tears during the funeral service and felt guilty for it. I'm pretty sure this makes me the worst person in the world. I still felt so stunned and numb that the service just seemed surreal and improper; like simply going through the motions of something, but I couldn't put my finger on what. Midway through, the funeral director, looking as if he partook of his own embalming fluid, warbled a song without musical accompaniment and I almost laughed out loud. His loud, opera-like voice echoed around the small chapel, too large for the space.

Mom, are you listening to this nonsense? This guy's hilarious. I looked around to see if anyone else considered the singing as ridiculous as I did, but most people were looking down or dabbing at their eyes.

Somebody had chosen old photographs to display of my mom, although I never found out who had taken this responsibility, and staring at them seemed almost absurd. Three family members stood up and spoke, telling loving stories that I had no recollection of, while an old friend of mine from high school sat beside me and gently rubbed my back. Katrina, still so young and unaware of the significance of the service, played obliviously in the back of the room with a couple of cousins and other children who came with family friends. She had a great time. A wooden box, meant to resemble a coffin, formed the center of everything, which I thought silly considering my mother was probably already just a pile of ash by this point. I kept thinking about the fact that I would have no place to go to visit my mother after today. My family had forever changed.

\*\*\*

I spent the remainder of the summer trying to keep myself busy, to give my life a semblance of normalcy and to help with the family finances. My dad encountered difficulty with his job search, which had begun before my mom's death and now entered its third month. He spent much of his time alone during the day. He always seemed a bit too excited to see me upon my return home from going out. Apparently feeling like he could not act as a very good father for the moment, he often sent my sister to a neighbor's house for the afternoon. I believed he couldn't stand the idea of Katrina having to see her father cry all of the time. Mickey must have begun to feel overwhelmed with all of the grief constantly encircling him, because he took the opportunity to buy a house down the street, and passed the current rental to my dad, to help make one less obstacle for the man who had lost his wife.

Meanwhile I lost all semblance of rational thought about my health. I constantly felt tingling in my arms and chest, maintained a steady level of nausea and fought crushing headaches on a daily basis. A parent of an old friend took me in for a couple of days and in order to calm my fears, invited me to see a cardiologist; the most established, reputable cardiologist in town. He performed an EKG on me and declared me tremendously healthy. I didn't believe him. So this friend's parent paid to send me to an expensive therapist, who listened to me cry and told me I wasn't going to die, at least now, from the causes I suspected; mainly, congestive heart failure. Or a heart attack of any kind. I received my first prescription for Xanax and Paxil. Against my father's wishes, I took the Xanax.

"That's for old people with real problems, not for young ladies," he said. He was mad and I was confused about why he thought anxiety drugs only worked for old people. And wasn't this situation a real problem? To me, this was the poster child of real problems. This whole period goes down in my history as my Blue Period. Only I don't have the fantastic art, like Van Gogh, to coincide with this designation.

\*\*\*

I arrived at the duplex one afternoon to see my father folded up on the couch facing the wall. At first I thought I had found him asleep, but then I heard sniffling and gently walked up to him, resting my hand on his shoulder. He flinched slightly but didn't acknowledge me with any words.

"Dad," I said. "What's going on? Are you feeling okay?" He just nodded and made a weak gesture with his visible arm to attempt to shoo me away. "Listen, I've been thinking. What if maybe I put off law school for a semester? Just temporarily. I can defer until January. Just so you can get back on your feet." I paused to see if he had any reaction. He continued to lay there, unmoved.

"Dad, you need help with Katrina and I can't stand the thought of leaving you guys like this." I swallowed, not wanting to say my next words, but knowing I needed to say them. "I can get a job and help earn some money to pay bills and keep us going. You shouldn't have to face all of this alone. It's not fair to you. And how is Katrina going to be once this really sinks in and she starts to understand what's going on and the permanence of it all? What do you think?" I reached in to touch his shoulder again.

He bolted up, a look of rage brewing in his eyes, causing me to startle. "Absolutely not! I will not tolerate you sacrificing your life for this. Your mother would have wanted you to keep going. It would've destroyed her to think that you would put your life on hold, jeopardize your future to stay home. And for what? She's not ever coming back. What good would you do here, in this, this place?" he asked, gesturing around the tiny, worn apartment. "Forget it. I'm having a rough time, yes, but that doesn't mean that I won't get through it. I'm a grown man and I don't need you hanging around here trying to 'take care of me.' And I don't want you worrying about me all of the time either. I'll find a job and I'll carry on and so will you."

"What about Katrina?" I asked, concerned.

"She'll be just fine. It's my top priority to make sure of it." As he looked at me, I could see the despondent haggardness behind his fiery facade, wanting to believe what he said but knowing the road ahead would prove much more difficult than his words suggested. "You're going up to Vermont at the end of August just like you're scheduled to do so that you can go to law school and make us proud. And I'm taking you there myself."

"I just thought…" I began, but then I saw the proud look in my father's eyes and backed down. "Okay," I said. Three weeks later, my father drove up to the front driveway with a borrowed pick-up truck so that he could drive me and my stuff all the way up the east coast.

Hypochondriac Lesson #12:

Taking a risk might just give you extra courage.

*12- Sex, Skunks and Palpitations*

Well, hello, there, Handsome. I had just stepped out of my room to take some yogurt to the common room fridge when I saw him. He smiled, I smiled and I retracted back into my room like a turtle. Smooth. I peeked back out of the door and it looked like he'd done the same double-take maneuver. Nice. His smile lit up the otherwise dim, old, wallpaper-peeling hallway; a hallway resembling that in "The Shining." I fully expected to see freaky twin girls or even a kid on a little tricycle down that hallway on any given night. But back to his smile. If we starred in a toothpaste commercial a little light would have twinkled on one of his teeth, while a cutesy bell sounded. Like Madeline Kahn singing "Oh sweet mystery of life I've found you," after having sex with the monster in "Young Frankenstein," I felt something. Magnetism. The earth moving. Love at first sight, perhaps? Let's say I had a different reaction than ever before.

I lived in a room in a turn-of-the-century inn turned law school dormitory, on the town green of a small town in Vermont, my home for my first year of law school. I had moved in a week before, with complete apprehension. I went from people to cows. I went from Blockbuster to the town movie rental shed. I don't think it had a name, and it was literally the size of a large closet, made of wood, and had no air conditioning. The New Releases rack, not a section or a wall, but a rack, held about ten movies. The rest of the movies derived from 1985, or an earlier vintage. And yet, it still had a curtained off doorway to a room the area of a smaller closet which held the adult videos. I never went in there, but always suspected they involved cows (animals, not large people). When my father drove me into this town, previously unseen by me, and well, most of the general population, I started to cry. What had I gotten myself into? Where would I eat?

Who would I talk to? Were there any stores anywhere? I didn't even see a gas
station. Oh, this could not be good. I could surely benefit from living a quieter
life with decreased stress, but this qualified as REMOTE.

It took a good four hours after arriving in town before I even saw a single
person outside of the Resident Advisor of the inn/dorm. Relief flooded through
me like a tsunami to even have met her. She assured me and my dad, who had,
by this point, also started questioning the reasonableness of leaving me in such a
sparse location, that I would find people to meet and places to eat, and a couple of
bars to drink. She whispered this last part to me. Only twenty-five minutes away,
I could find a real grocery store and slew of great restaurants like Friendly's. Well,
if there's a Friendly's, I guess I'd have to stay for three years and see this thing
through. She did, however, direct us to a little breakfast shack about five rural
miles away, where I savored my first portion of real Vermont maple syrup and eggs
smothered in Vermont cheddar cheese. The meal changed my mind. I figured I
could stick it out after that. I felt full of pancakes and hope.

I moved in first but once others started arriving to fill the Inn and its fifteen
rooms, I realized I might actually have a chance to form a little community. As
the cars drove in to town and graced the small law school campus, I met them
before I met the people who owned them. Lots of wagons, Subarus, old Volvos
and my favorite, an old white Merkur littered with twenty to thirty bumper
stickers celebrating every liberal cause you can possibly imagine. Hug a bunny. Go
Abortion! Rainbow flags, Save the World and all its components, it takes a village,
love not guns. I mean the owner of this car CARED. And didn't discriminate in the
caring and loving. For a few days, I didn't know who possessed this car, but every
day that I passed it, on the way back from the post office, or bookstore, I tried to
read at least one new bumper sticker. I couldn't help admiring the passion present

to warrant defacing a perfectly undented automobile. Then I met the him. And his smile shined a warm light on my dark mind which had grown cold with grief and fear.

Jason.

I'm not quite sure why he fell for me. Let's face it. I was a complete mess. I cried all the time as my mother's death still bled fresh; less than two months old. And now, I ventured into brand new territory; new state, new school, new chapter of my life. All of which would have been nerve wracking enough, but add my undying sadness to the mix and I struggled to make it through the night. Those wee hours weren't going so well. I woke every single night, without exception, at 1:30 a.m., the same time my father had wakened me when my mother lost her life; and never quite managed to fall back to sleep until the safety of the sun started to emerge. Then I felt comfortable to drift until my alarm went off shortly thereafter. My body had lost a great deal of weight, so maybe my thin frame attracted him. I certainly cannot credit the dark circles under my eyes. Happily enough, I loved my hair at this time. Normally, my dark, thick, ropy, unruly natural curls twisted, waved and drifted in various layers of frizz in the humidity of the south. But here, the hair angels sang. With the drier air, I had a gorgeous, if temporary, mane of perfectly aligned S-waves; if I do say so myself. So maybe the hair drew him to me. Whatever it was, I am eternally grateful.

Jason, with the dark olive green eyes, heavy shiny brown hair, even heavier eyelashes, and lips that never needed chapstick. He turned my bluest days into days of discovery, laughter, and thoughtfulness. Sure, I would've made it through the tragedy and big changes in my life eventually, if not clumsily. I have that fight in me. But I can say definitively that he made the experience a LOT easier to endure. And I felt the difference from the moment I first beheld that smile. It took less than a week to consider this guy the ultimate guy for me.

We started to explore the area before school started, to get to know each other and the other students, and prepare for our first law school classes. Five of us from the Inn decided to take a day and really see Vermont as a Vermonter. We went hiking. Jason, an avid outdoorsy fellow, picked the location. A mountain called Camel's Hump, about forty-five minutes through the Green Mountains from our little town of South Royalton. As we drove, I marveled at the beauty of the landscape; how the clouds hovered over the tops of the mountains like whipped cream on a perfectly served sundae, drips of which clung further down the side, while clear blue filled the rest of the sky. I wanted to stick my head out of the window like a Golden Retriever so I could more deeply inhale the smell of the mist on the lush green trees; such a pure, clean, natural scent, like grass and flowers right after a rainstorm. With no billboards to block the view, a state law, we became part of the landscape instead of just passersby.

Once we arrived at the parking area to commence the hike, however, the tension start tweaking the muscles in my chest. What if I wasn't physically capable of climbing this mountain? I looked around at the height of the peaks and tried not to note that our destination was listed as taller than those in my immediate view. What if I injured myself? What if I had a heart attack on the way up, or at the top? I would die, because they couldn't get me to the emergency room in time. And where the heck was the emergency room, anyway? I hadn't seen a hospital anywhere in this state. I could feel the panic coming on and I started shaking out my hands. I will not die this way. I repeated it to myself like a mantra.

"Are you okay?" Jason asked me. Apparently, my face gave me away.

"What? Oh, me?" I feigned innocence. Like, oh please, I'm as cool as a cucumber, happy as a clam, easy as Sunday Morning; you name the cliché. "I'm great. Just excited to tackle this mountain," I said with a "can-do" attitude. I would not show him my true nature at this point. I couldn't allow him to see the sheer enormity of my craziness; not yet. I knew the impossibility of always hiding it, but might as well create the illusion that I was a cool girl, not afraid of anything. Complaining about heart troubles, brain tumors, passing out, etc. might put a damper on our budding relationship. But to put it mildly, I felt like my organs had started to turn inside out and bits of them might sputter out of all of my orifices. Remember, I lived in Florida all my life. I'd never hiked anything taller than a landfill (don't ask). I've summited tall mountains in Switzerland, but rode to the top on a train. I attended camp in North Carolina, but the hikes stayed fairly conservative since we were a bunch of eleven-year-old girls, carrying our own stuff. My parents did not hike. Not once. Ever. So the task ahead seemed rather daunting to me. I had to put my trust in Jason, in that smile. And have faith in myself. Oy.

We started the climb, and after the initial despair that my heart might give out on me as it beat so very fast, I found myself developing a bit of a rhythm. Jason had directed me to a large stick to use as a hiking pole and I began to rather enjoy myself. Sure, I had quite a bit of trouble catching my breath, especially keeping up with the rest of the group who had apparently hiked all their lives. At least three of them harbored fantasies of climbing Mount Everest. For me, today would be my Mount Everest. I would conquer this mountain and hopefully my fears; of heights, of wide open spaces, of dying. A big moment, surely. I decided to take it slowly, and enjoy the trees and nature all around me. I found myself asking questions about the flora and fauna and Jason would always give up the lead to backtrack and answer my questions. I must have resembled an eager Girl Scout. Or teacher's pet. But he didn't seem to mind. In fact, he allowed the others to continue forward while he stayed in the back with me. I pretended I wanted to take in all the grandeur and awe-inspiring beauty, but truthfully I couldn't keep up with the pace. Lame, I know.

Four to five hours later; that's right, folks, it took us that long of hiking up, just to get near the top; we exited the tree line (a "line" I did not formerly know to exist until right at this moment) and suddenly we had to scramble over rocks. Where did the trail go? Oh my god! It just disappeared. I crouched down on all fours like a cheetah; but oh, not fast at all. Rather, my hands slapped down instinctively to get me closer to the ground as quickly as possible. I could see all around, a perfect, unfiltered view for miles of all the mountains. Quite a sight. I thought I might throw up from the magnitude of it all.

"Is there enough oxygen up here?" I asked, gasping for air and not quite filling my lungs. Great. A collapsed lung. Hadn't thought of that one yet today.

"That's funny," Jason said, clearing thinking I jested. Then, seeing me blinking furiously and starting to wonder why I stayed on all fours, he said, "We're really not high enough for that kind of thing." I noticed the perplexed arch of his eyebrow. Uh oh. I couldn't give myself away. Stand up, Kat! You're already up here. Now act like a normal human being. Enjoy the view, for crying out loud.

I coolly rose and brushed off my knees. No sense holding on to the dirty reminder of my fear. I walked across that bald mountain, considering the trees encircling it as a shameless hairline, providing false pretenses to the actual state of the coverage. Mean trees, deceiving me that way. But okay, fair enough. The vertigo crept over me as I looked around. I didn't see much to protect me if I fell. I knew it would end in certain demise. I looked down at my cheap, Payless, yellow worker boots that I currently tried to pass off as hiking boots, and cursed them. Plus a painful stinging feeling had started to take over my heels. I found a large boulder to sit on and untied my shoe. I shrieked; which I'm sure echoed off the mountains like an out of control boomerang; when my eyes rested on the large circular pad of a puss-filled blister that ballooned off the back of my heel. I winced as I touched it. Curiosity got the better of me; killed the Kat, if you will. No? Fine. Unable to stand the sight of blood or anything painful, I groaned and felt the wooziness wash over me. Not a nice combination with vertigo, I can tell you.

Within half a second, Jason found his spot by my side and had already unzipped his backpack and pulled out his first aid kit. Who needs a doctor in the house when you've got this guy?

He quickly assessed the problem and then worked on cutting a piece of mole skin to fit over the blister and protect it from further irritation. He applied it to my skin, holding my foot delicately, while down on one knee, like the prince putting the glass slipper on Cinderella. He reached further into his bag and pulled out an extra pair of hiking socks- yes, there are differences between regular socks and good hiking socks- and told me to wear them over my other socks to reduce the rubbing on my heel. Once I put all layers and my cheapo boots back on, I felt instant relief. I looked at him with awe, like he was a hero, or MacGyver. I did not know boys like these growing up. Where did he come from? Where had he been all my life? Surprisingly, in Florida, where he, too, had grown up and lived. We discussed places of common interest in the sunshine state over our packed lunches on that rocky mountaintop and I felt myself start to relax. I had to admit, we had an unbeatable view for dining on trail mix, granola bars and PB&J's. Maybe there was something to this whole hiking thing. After about thirty minutes, the group decided to head back down, as we didn't want to get stuck hiking the trail after dark. I heartily agreed; could not agree more. With renewed interest in the outdoors, I threw my backpack on my back and followed the crew over the bald rocks to continue the trail that would lead down.

A few minutes later I found myself facing a unique arrangement in order to progress down the "trail" (at this particular spot, that term could not have applied, as the "trail" did not have width enough to stand with both feet side-by-side). By all accounts, this spot required the designation of "cliff", or "sheer, heart-stopping drop off." But certainly not "trail." I stood rooted to my current boulder. I thought about revisiting my four-legged crouch, but wasn't sure about next steps after that. Jason, already on the other side of the area, turned to make sure I made it.

"You just kind of need to shimmy," he said.

"Shimmy?" I asked.

"Yeah, just put your left foot there. Keep your back up against the rocks and just…shimmy across." Right, shimmy. No problem. Piece of freakin' cake.

I stepped my left foot out, pressed my back as far against the rock as possible, considering that the blasted backpack caused me to bow outward at the chest. If I could have melted into that rock, I would have. I brought my right foot on the ledge to join the rest of me and spread my arms out, eagle style, to grasp the rocks behind me. Okay, done. Then I looked out. Oh no. I can't breathe. Can't. Catch. My. Breath. Don't look down. Don't look down. Shit. I just looked down and there is nothing. If I fall, the first tree available will kill me. Why did I do this? Why am I here? This is not me. I don't belong here. I must be out of my mind!

I have since labeled this moment as "Precipice Paralysis." The visible elements of my body stayed frozen while my organs went on autopilot with the dial set at "Haywire." My heart raced at a pace unmatched in previous circumstances. If I didn't fall, I knew this would end me. And clearly the lack of breathing would take its toll anytime. The swooshing in my ears turned me deaf. It took a while (seconds? Minutes? Hours?) before I realized Jason was actually trying to communicate with me. I peered over at him, slowly, trying to avoid any sudden movements. He had reached his arm out to me and seemed to say something about stepping.

"Take your left foot and step about one foot to the left with it." I mutely obeyed. "Now take your right foot and pull it to meet up with your left." Okay, check. I could not move otherwise. "Now do that two more times. And keep holding on to the rock as you slide over. You're doing great, Kat." Not really. But okay. Believing you seems to help. "Now take your right foot and try to put it right on this groove here on this rock. It kind of looks like a shelf. If you can put your foot there and give me your hand, I can pull you up. Okay?" I took the order and followed his instructions. And you know what? I made it. As I found my footing, that is, both feet securely on solid boulder ground, where no little pebbles would slip and fall silently into the abyss below until a faint sound might emanate from the bottom, an enormous gust of air pushed its way out of my lungs so that my breathing sputtered back to life. I gasped. I heaved. I might have thrown up a little. But I made it. We started heading back toward the beloved tree line, that safe haven of blocked views, and I felt sublime. I climbed a mountain and my heart raced and I lost my breath and I might have slipped to my death, but I escaped alive. The others barely acknowledged the ledge, but to me, I had triumphed over adversity, triumphed over my own doubt. With the help of handy step-by-step instructions, sure. But I like to think that I would've shimmied on my own if I had traveled alone.

That night, and about five days after, my legs turned to jelly and then harbored the sorest muscles I have ever encountered in all of my existence. More than any dancing or cheerleading, or walking, or running, or anything ever caused me. The pain lit my thighs on fire and if I tried to do something daring like sit, or stand up from a sitting position, my legs protested, my eyes teared up, and I exclaimed openly, and often rudely. Like a ninety-year old man who's been idle for decades, I could hardly move. I seriously considered inquiring after a walker. My third floor room did not aid in pain reduction, as the steep stairs served as my nemeses during this agonizing period. I experienced such all encompassing soreness, that I had trouble stepping into the tub and twice bungled my attempts to do just that, causing excruciating bruises on my shins from hitting the side of the bathtub. Sad, really. And more than a little embarrassing.

Oh, and the night before classes began, we got skunked.

I should explain. See, Vermonters don't typically have air conditioning. Raised in Florida, I simply do not understand this method of living. Why tolerate heat, when you can see your breath inside? I cherish the idea of snuggling underneath my down comforter even if the thermometer outside reads ninety-six degrees. Vermonters figure that summers don't last too long, so air conditioning just wastes money. All I know is that those first few weeks at the end of summer, before fall blessed us with coolness and radiant color, we sweltered. I blasted three fans on me at once while I slept under the thinnest sheet. I kept both of my windows open in hopes of a pittance of air circulation, to no avail. I suffered for this. One night, the power went out (a whisper threw the power out in that area, so this was not uncommon or unexpected, even if we detected no looming storm on the horizon). Around midnight, the earth stood still. My fans warbled into a slow death. The air halted completely and I heard nothing. Then, the most satanic sound I have ever heard emanated from the hills. Arguably, I have not really heard any other satanic sounds, but trust me, this is what I imagined Satan sounding like.

"Mwahhhhhh," said the eerie ghost, the whimper echoing off the quiet, yet receptive, mountains. "Ahhhhhhh. Rahhhhhhh. Mwahhhrrrr."

I leapt out of my bed, understanding that I would encounter the "Shining" moment I'd been expecting since arrival in the hallway. Phew. Surprisingly all clear. I tore into Jason's room, without politely knocking to waken him. I shook him awake.

"Come quick! It's the devil." His eyes widened out of sleep. If I looked closely, I could probably see his heart beat through the sheets. In hindsight, I realize I might have chosen a gentler approach of bringing the demonic noise to his attention. But truth told, I wanted to fling myself behind his armoire and hide until morning. The sun always drove the demons away, right?

"What are you talking about?" he asked, but still jumped out of bed, scuffling around to find some clothes to put on, ready to humor me even in this most ridiculous of circumstances.

"Just come with me. I don't know what it is, but it's freaking me out. It's right by my window." We raced down to the other end of the hall to my room and then stood in the middle of the room to wait for the noise. Still. Silent. Fools.

"Mwahhhhrrr. Ahhhhhhhr."

"See? There! Listen." The noise sounded again, this time louder and closer. Jason walked to the window. I tried to grab him. Please don't go! I don't want the monsters to get you. Then he cracked up. He started laughing so hard that he had to sit down on my bed. I politely laughed along, so he wouldn't feel stupid. He could hardly speak.

"Oh, Kat, you're so funny. The Devil!" He started laughing again.

"Yeah, so what's so funny?"

"Your devils are some horny cats. Must be mating season."

"What? Are you kidding me?" I bolted over to the window for a better look. One window overlooked the railroad tracks, video shack and a cemetery on a hill (a tough image to swallow at first when I arrived), and the other window overlooked the downstairs pub and dumpster. At first I didn't see the coquettish animals in question. Then they sounded their love call and I followed the noise with my eyes until I saw the dirty deed. "Oh my god! Is he killing her?" Jason just laughed some more.

"They'll be fine. And so will you. Are you okay now that you know that the gates of hell haven't opened outside your window? I'm really tired and think I might head back to bed."

"Yeah, sure. Go ahead. I'm sorry I woke you." I waved him off to disregard the incident. "You have to admit, though, that was one scary sound." I said this to his back as he walked down the hallway. He turned around and blew a kiss at me. Sigh.

But back to the skunks. So, the night before classes started, we all went to bed, nervous and excited with anticipation. We had read our first assignments, busily taking notes on everything so that we could survive the Socratic Method in Contracts class the next day. We knew, and had heard tear-laced horror stories, of how the law school professors called on one or two unsuspecting students and painfully grilled them the whole class. Almost weekly, a woefully unprepared student would flee the scene, shaken and emotional from the hurricane force battering of his or her memory and reasoning skills. Academic brutality. Since we were not really familiar with the proceedings aside from these cryptic tales, we were scared. We tossed and turned. And we got skunked.

Around six a.m. in the morning, I woke to a most horrific odor. I could almost see the hue of the stench in the air, clinging to my Kmart drapes and flirting with my comforter. I coughed and my eyes watered for protection. Could I be having a seizure? Didn't a person experience phantom smells from strokes and seizures? I quickly went to the bathroom, ran a shower and got in, squirting more than my usual allotment of soap and shampoo onto my body, as insurance against THAT smell. My windows had remained open throughout the night and the smell materialized everywhere. I couldn't escape it. I ventured back into my room and it had intensified since I'd tried to erase my memory of it with bottled scents. I opened up my closets, thinking that if I could just dress quickly and head out to class, and probably eat breakfast at a town café (because who really could have an appetite with that grotesqueness wafting around), I could air out and put the whole nasty business behind me. I grabbed my books and backpack and scurried out the door like the large striped vermin who had caused this affliction in the first place.

I settled into my chosen chair in class and waited for others to arrive. As I perused my notes, I saw the next class member arrive. In an attempt to be friendly, he sat a couple of chairs over from me, so we could discuss the assignment. After about thirty seconds, the smile disappeared from his face and he looked like he might vomit.

"Are you nervous about the professor?" I asked, in my friendliest, most neighborly way. I relaxed back into my chair, rocking back and forth on its legs, in a most confident fashion. "I wouldn't worry about it. You did the reading, right? And besides, there're like fifty people in the class. Chances are, you won't even be up today." I smiled.

"Um, yeah. Nervous. In fact, I think I better go sit over there and study a little more before everyone arrives." He quickly retreated to the far corner of the room, on the opposite side from me. Man, these kids are high strung. What's the worst that can happen if you get called on?

Jason arrived next with two other Inn dwellers and they all happily sat down around me. We had bonded over that hike and already numerous dinners and quaint get-to-know-you chats while watching endless repeats of Law and Order, a law student staple. We were the little law student family at the Inn. Very special. I almost wanted to hug them as a group. Others must have been intimidated by our unity, because as they entered, if they sat near us, they soon exited our vicinity and gravitated to the other side of the room. Finally the professor arrived and everyone settled into fevered silence. The inhabitants of the room made a few final coughs and throat clearings. The professor looked up and pretended to notice for the first time that he now stood in front of a room full of people. He looked from one side to the other, and then furrowed his brow.

"Is there a reason why there are only five people on the left side of the room and everyone else on the right side of the room? I don't think I've ever seen that before. Usually it's more in the back and only Kiss Asses in the front." A few people in the front row shifted uncomfortably in their seats. A student on the other side of the room, the full side, raised his hand. "Yes?"

"If I may, Professor, it's because it really stinks over there. Like skunk." He pointed at us accusingly. Oh my god! I'm the one that smells. We are a group that smells and now that is how everyone will now remember us. Including this man that will grade my exam. Are people prejudiced against those who smell? Do they have greeting cards for this kind of thing? Our little group collectively laughed uncomfortably, all of us as bright red as a British man on the coast of Spain on summer vacation.

"I see." He looked at us with amusement. "Very well, then. Let's move on. You, sir...your name is?" He directed his question at the accuser. "You get to be on the hot seat today."

Sweet justice. I'll always love that man, my contracts professor. I guess he figured that getting skunked was enough shame for one day and he saved his chance to disgrace us further until another class hour. The accuser left the building that day, feeling as bad as we smelled. It took us days and professional cleaning to get the odor out of all of our clothes, hair and linens. Dastardly little critters, those skunks. They happened to live right outside my window, right by the dumpster. I liked to imagine that they talked like Pepe Le Pew and courted each other, experiencing the very first signs of love, like me. It was the only way I could tolerate them.

    \*\*\*

My romance with Jason escalated quickly after we met. Once you've summited an impressive mountain and had the good fortune of sharing a decent skunking, love seemed like the logical next step. Turns out, I was right on the money. He shaved his beard, because he heard on some late night talking extravaganza fueled by chillable red Franzia, the boxed wine, that I hated facial hair. We kissed the next day. A couple of weeks later, we were snuggling after watching a video, enjoying the cool fall air breezing in, and oops, we had sex. Funny how that worked out. I mean, I'd waited for so long, and then, like nothing out of the ordinary, boom. Done deal. For once, I didn't worry if I was making a bad decision. Everything just seemed right, somehow. I had no doubts whatsoever. Twenty-one years old. Hard to believe. But those are the facts. Everything had fallen into place, despite the tragedy, despite my fears, despite the darkness. For one small instant, I thought maybe my worries would all disappear. That was a good moment.

But like all good hypochondriacs, it was only a matter of time. I laugh at my naiveté.

Hypochondriac Lesson #13:
Try a different doctor; like a therapist.

## 13- Crash and Sizzle Like Bacon

Don't ever let anyone tell you that law school isn't adventurous. Early one Tuesday morning, the first week of April during my premier year at that fine institution, the phone startled me awake as it rang ominously from the other side of the room. Who could be calling me at this time of day? Certainly nobody who knows me very well. Frankly, not many people called these days. Outside of the small circle of friends in the school, I had morphed into a hermit for my studies.

I reached out and mumbled an irritated "hullo" into the receiver, not even sure that I spoke into the right end of the thing.

"Kathleen, is that you?"

"Who's this?" I asked, thinking that I sort of recognized the voice but just couldn't place it. Nobody but family ever referred to me by my full name.

"Kathleen, this is your Uncle." He paused. "How're you doing up there in New England? Surviving the cold?"

I wrinkled up my face in consternation. Was this man really calling me this early in the morning to make small talk? To discuss the northern weather? Then I realized that made no sense at all and suddenly felt fully awake. My stomach dropped to the floor, as if riding a double-looped roller coaster. I answered his questions with one or two words, then held my breath and waited for the chandelier of his words to crash dramatically to the floor, Phantom of the Opera style.

"Kathleen, I'm calling about your father." He hesitated and I could hear his nervous intake of breath. "He's in the hospital." I reached out to grab a pillow and hold it to my chest as a reactionary comfort. My heart shambled into an irregular beat and I felt the last vestiges of stability escape me. Had I not been sitting, I would have fallen. I didn't want bad news, but sensed it coming, like a dog senses a bad storm hours before arrival. "Last night he was eating dinner, apparently with some friends and starting having chest pains and a hard time breathing. Stubborn as he is, he didn't want anyone to make a big fuss about it and tried to go on eating. You know how he likes to eat." I winced. "But finally his friends convinced him that he needed to go to the hospital. His color looked pretty bad, so he finally went. They drove him because he wouldn't tolerate them calling an ambulance." He paused to chuckle over my dad's audacity, but then stopped himself at the inappropriateness of laughter at this particular time. "Your dad's had a heart attack and while he's okay since they caught it in time, they're going to have to do open heart surgery. Triple bypass is what they told me."

A startled sob escaped from my lips. You've got to be fucking kidding me! Forget my stupid cussing rules. Hadn't my family been through enough already? What gives? I somehow managed to utter words to the effect of needing to make travel plans. I felt horrible for thinking of practicalities, but how was I supposed to get away and still finish the semester with strong grades? If I missed classes, I wouldn't catch up to perform well on the finals. I couldn't blow these off. Had someone placed a curse on me when I wasn't looking? Did I tick off some voodoo witch the last time I was in New Orleans? My karma must be extremely poor. I must have done all sorts of crazy things in a former life. Then my stomach dropped again, skidding the bottom, as I had another thought. What about Katrina? She was six years old, for crying out loud. She already dealt with more crap than any other little girl her age. Uncle interrupted my frantic thought track.

"He doesn't want you to come down."

"What do you mean? Of course I have to go down there. He can't do this alone. He can't be by himself. I'm his daughter and I have to be there to help him get through this." I felt my body tensing by the second and my voice elevated in pitch to where I bordered sounding hysterical; like a panicked cheerleader.

"Kathleen, listen, I know this is hard for you, but he doesn't want you there. He thinks it would be harder to go into surgery if he had to look at you beforehand. He believes that this way he can pretend it's just something else that he has to do. He has to live because he has your sister relying on him and needing him to survive."

"But..."

"He said if there are a lot of people around, crying and all that, he would feel more like he is about to die. That scares him more. At least this way, he's not questioning whether he will make it. He's just expecting to. And honestly, I'm inclined to agree with him. Do you understand?"

I nodded my head slowly, resignedly, only realizing moments later that I needed to say something as he could not see the movement of my head.

"I understand," I said as I tried to contain my crying. I'm not usually a big crier. But I had shed more tears since my mother died than I had in all the years of my life up to this point, combined. I thought maybe I had started to dry up, like an old well. And now this. My father had a point.

"Kathleen, I'll be down there, and I'll call you each step of the way so that you'll know what's going on. But more than anything I want you to try not to worry." Fat chance. He didn't know me too well. "He wants you to stay up there and focus on your studies, okay?" His constant use of my name disconcerted me. I assumed that he had repeated it as a way to ground me, keep my terror more earthbound, instead of letting it all fly wild into the stratosphere and explode like fireworks with color and vividness. He did not succeed. I felt like I was tied to the back of a speedboat and was painfully bouncing and crashing around in rough water with no sight of land.

I waited by the phone the entire next day, knowing that my father would enter surgery around ten in the morning. The doctors said the surgery would take four to five hours and that once he made it through, he would reside in the ICU for at least a day before I could to talk with him. I urgently wanted to hear in his voice that he'd made it out of the woods. I skipped my Civil Procedure class and hoped that a kind soul would take pity on me and share notes. All day I paced my room thinking of my sister. How could a six-year-old girl lose her father only a couple of months after losing her mother? Such a bad fate rearing its unbearable head on innocence made no sense. Maybe bad things just happen sometimes.

As usual, my mind reached for the worst-case scenario. What if he died? How would I take care of my sister? I lived in a room, with a shared bathroom for the whole floor. I walked in on naked people all the time. I hadn't even finished my first year of law school. I had a new boyfriend who would most certainly want to high tail it out of my life rather than deal with this burden. I had no idea where to even begin. I needed to stop thinking about it and hope for the best. My heart couldn't bear another choice. It had other issues to deal with, like constant palpitations. At certain moments a beat would strike so hard I thought a gong had sounded in my chest. It hurt; never a good sign. If my mother could die from heart disease, and my father needed triple bypass surgery for heart disease, then I was doomed. Plus he had the diabetes problem. Man, my genes went progressively south on an annual basis.

As three o'clock that afternoon rolled around, I still hadn't heard from Uncle. My stomach toiled and reeled within me but I tried to breathe deeply; a tough job considering that each breath felt like a stretch, a thick rubber band inside my lungs that required more muscle than I could muster. I reached into my brain to dig out the teensy bit of yoga information I could find, from a video I had watched once, to try to calm my frazzled nerves and just steady myself. I don't think I had much success. All I could remember was Downward Dog (not helpful to have a rush of blood to my head at the moment) and Corpse Pose (really didn't want to engage in that ill named pose at all). I could only focus on the phone and how hard my heart beats felt. At four, just as I bit my last nail down to the quick, drawing a small bubble of blood, my phone rang.

"Kathleen, he made it through," he blurted out with clear relief. He sounded as he if was releasing his own fear with the expulsion of the words from his lips.

"Oh thank God," I said. "What did the doctors say? I started to get worried because it seemed to be taking longer than what you said they thought it would take." Did that even make sense?

"Well, once they got into the surgery, they realized that another main artery was blocked and they needed to conduct a fourth bypass. But they caught it and said this should make him feel much better. It's just the recovery time can be kind of long on these things. He's not going to feel really great for at least six weeks and he can't lift anything over five pounds for the first three weeks."

"Wow, how's he going to do that? I mean who's going to take care of him? My sister's only six, for God's sake!"

"I know, I know. It's so hard. But your dad's been making friends down here and he's gotten involved in a church and, well, you wouldn't believe how many people have called me to offer help. There's one woman who's a retired nurse who's offered to go and stay with them for the first couple of weeks at least. And it's like people have started divvying up tasks, like who's going to bring food on what day and who's going to come by to clean." He started chuckling. "I mean it's pretty amazing. I don't know if it's because they know he's a single dad with a little girl or if he's just charming as hell to these people, but by God, I've never seen anything like it."

I sat on the edge of my bed, stunned. There seemed to be so much that I didn't know about my father's life. I reminisced about how I felt in those last few weeks of my mother's life, when she had started sharing stories about her childhood that I'd never heard before, like she knew the end loomed. How could I live with my parents for eighteen years and miss so much of their personalities and histories? I felt ashamed; my family seemed slightly alien to me at the moment. I also experienced great relief that I'd been spared from having to take care of my sister, at least for now. I wondered if my relief would have disappointed my father.

"Thank you, Uncle. Thank you for taking care of him, being with him when he needed it like that. It means so much to me. But also, thank you for telling me about his friends." I smiled through the quiet tears running from my eyes, down the side of my nose. More of the darn crying? Is there an endless supply, because I'm sure I must be close to the edge of mine otherwise?

"You know, I really think he's going to be okay. Now I want to know that you're going to be okay, too." I laughed openly, even though he would never truly understand why.

"I'm certainly going to give it my best shot." If I don't fall down dead from the heart attack I think I'm having right now.


"Which way do I go now?" I asked myself aloud in the car. I always talk to myself. Maybe I enjoy my own company. I do crack myself up sometimes. But that's good, right? You can't be interesting to other people if you find yourself uninteresting. That's the theory I'm going with to justify talking to myself. Other drivers have been privy to the show and I'm sure they've laughed at me, but oh well.

I had purchased a car down south right before law school, a dark red Dodge Neon (not candy apple red, but a darker, more dignified shade), that I'd named Lumiere and my father called "Puff", short for Strawberry Cream Puff. The time limit to register the car in my new state approached. I decided to skip out on a criminal law class- according to these tales, I skipped class all the time, but I really didn't; I promise- to take the car over to the state police station for the inspection required in order to receive a Vermont license plate. I hated these kinds of errands. My father always handled this kind of stuff for my mother, so maybe I thought it was 'Man's Work.' I also knew that life without a car in this rural area of the world would be pretty unbearable. I wound my way on narrow roads towards the police station - actually a double-wide trailer located in a small town nearby; pretty advanced architecture for those entrusted to keep us safe. As I'd never driven that way before (this preceded GPS systems), I pulled into the parking lot of an oddly located music school to get my bearings and make sure I did not miss my intended destination. After a minute of looking around, I spotted the trailer about half a mile down the road. Although the day shown sunny and clear, a recent snow had passed through the area and the snow plows had pushed large white snow drifts up on the sides of all the roads, making it difficult to see down each direction over the dirty white mini mountains.

I inched the car out slowly to make the left turn towards the station, while Def Leppard's "Pour Some Sugar on Me" kept me pumped for the occasion. Seeing nobody, I accelerated and continued across the road. The deafening noise of metal crunching metal took me completely by surprise and I let out a quick, and quite loud, scream as a large white mass smashed into my side of the car and sent me in a spin that ended in a ditch on the other side of the road. Oh my god! What just happened? Am I dead? Am I bleeding? Can I move? Why did my car sound like crumpling tin foil just now? I sat stunned and trembling for a minute trying to figure out if I were dead or alive. I fully expected to get out of the car and still see myself sitting there. All of the air vents and radio knobs had popped out of the dashboard and landed scattered on the seats and floor, but my radio still played the music as if nothing had happened. "*...I'm hot, sticky sweet, from my head, to my feet, Yeah!*" The air bag had deployed, hitting the side of my head, knocking the large, banana size, jaw clip out of my hair and through the back windows. I later found it on the ground, part of the casualties from an unexpected battle. All the inch-long teeth were still intact, but I could only image what that would have done to the back of my skull if I had not had my head turned. Talk about a headache! Or brain spillage. I looked up, still seated at this point, and saw what had been the white mass, now clearly a large white sedan, tilted off the road further up. I hoped to God that the person inside had lived through impact. Please don't be dead. Please don't be dead. I CANNOT have killed a person. Or people. Oh, just please be alive and okay. Did I mention that my father still recovered in the hospital from his bypass surgery? That's right, this little accident occurred only two days after my father went under the knife. That's good timing.

I got out of the car relatively easily, but noticed that my hands were swollen and bleeding and my legs had trouble holding me up and steady. I felt like a wooden puppet, when somebody lets go of the strings and it kind of wobbles back and forth, not standing, but not quite falling down either.

I dazedly looked around at the scene and noticed two or three women running towards me from the direction of the music school. They crossed the street to help me. I could see their young pupils standing in the doorway, one with a violin and the other with a horn of some kind. I wonder if they know Def Leppard? They had heard the impact from inside and now came to investigate. The state police arrived seconds later, coming just down the road. They probably witnessed the crash out of the windows of their offices, I remember thinking, ruefully. If I had to crash somewhere, at least it was convenient. And finally, I noticed the front door of the white car open slowly and a white-haired man of about seventy step out, all in one piece, thank the lord. He walked briskly over to me with worry imprinted all over his face.

"Miss, are you all right? I don't know how this happened. I didn't see you at all! And I know you couldn't have seen me. Are you injured? Oh, look at your hands." I just nodded and smiled weakly at him to let him know I was okay, but I couldn't find my words. I had witnessed accidents and fender benders before in Florida and nobody had ever been this nice about them. People usually threw their hands up in the air aggressively, while shouting blame at the other party. I loved Vermont more in that instant than I ever thought possible.

A state trooper stepped in and told me he would take me to the station and let me calm down and rest for a minute. Then he needed to take my statement.

"Are you sure you're okay?" he kept asking. "We can get you an ambulance if you think you need to go to the hospital."

"I don't have twelve hundred dollars!" I yelled. I didn't just pull this number out of thin air. The Florida ambulance that took my mother to her death at the hospital had sent us the bill for just this figure. I had no idea ambulances cost so much to use. The officer raised one eyebrow and appeared to analyze me quietly for a moment too long for my liking.

"Are you sure, Miss, that you don't need to see a doctor?" Geez, what is with this guy?

I muttered that I thought I was all right, maybe just a bit cut up and bruised.

When I got to the station, I excused myself and went to the bathroom to wash up a little bit and make sure I hadn't peed or soiled myself. I looked in the mirror. The pupils of my eyes were bigger than I'd ever seen them, like a cat ready to fight, and they weren't changing size with the light at all. I started to feel lightheaded and stepped back out into the office and told the officer to make the call to the hospital.

"I thought you might feel that way," he said, "so I already called the ambulance. They should be here any minute." Why didn't you tell me that I had no colored part of the eye left, you fool? It's all pupil! I looked feral. That's not normal. A funny mixture of fear and relief washed over me. The last person I knew who got into an ambulance never returned home. Certainly I couldn't be in that bad of shape. Would I be able to stomach seeing the interior of a vehicle I had so recently associated with death? When the ambulance arrived, the emergency workers escorted me to the back of the truck and I climbed in by myself and sat off to one side as if to still make room for someone on a stretcher. A female EMT hopped into the back with me and started taking my vital signs.

"I'm new and you're my first car accident," she said proudly with a big smile. I tried to smile back encouragingly but only managed to look slightly sick. The woman continued on, "You know, this ambulance is new and is actually the first one in a fifty mile radius. If you would've gotten in this wreck last week, we would've had to pick you up in a hearse. Heh heh." She could tell I found little humor in her anecdote, so she continued her procedure in silence. When faced with a brush with death, I didn't want to think about riding in the car that usually carries the dead. Today just wasn't turning out to be a good day.

"Hmm, that's weird," she said, as she held up my hand and pressed the tops of each of my fingernails individually. I wanted to smack her. Was she really just telling someone like me that my vital signs were "weird?" I must have some sort of internal injury from the accident. I will bleed internally and die. This is it. And only a few months after my mother and WHILE my father is still in the hospital recovering from a near-death experience. Okay, I needed to make some serious peace with God.

We arrived at the hospital and the EMT said, "Listen honey, my name is Charlene and I'm going to call you later on to make sure that you get home safely. I know you're scared but you're going to be just fine. I promise. I think you're just in a little bit of shock right now, that's all." She smiled warmly at me and gave my arm a slight squeeze as she handed me off to the emergency room attendant at the small hospital.

The uniformed attendant ushered me into a tiny, closet-sized space where a nurse drew an aquamarine curtain all the way around me to form a private room. I sat for a long time in that curtained off space that smelled like antiseptic and mop water. In fact, I started to find the wait kind of rude considering I'd been involved in a terrible car crash. By the way, what happened to my car? I just left it there on the side of the road. I had no idea what happened in these types of circumstances. I started fussing over my swollen hands. They had already begun to discolor, purple and yellow boundaries encircling the dried blood.

A commotion interrupted the otherwise strangely quiet emergency room. I had thought I occupied the whole ER by myself. But I heard all sorts of yelling and cussing and discussion about animals. I don't think most people share the same experience in other ERs around the country. Finally the doctor flung my curtain open, and stomped over to me, out of breath.

"Sorry about the wait. A man had a terrible accident with his pig." I just looked at her. What could that possibly mean? I didn't even want to attempt to guess the details. She didn't laugh when she said it, although I had trouble keeping a straight face, even through my injuries. A pig? Really? Now my car accident seemed wholly uninteresting.

Tall and pretty, the doctor had long dark hair and could not have exceeded age thirty-two. What circumstances had brought her here, to deal with Pig Boy and Snow Drift Accident Girl? Only in rural Vermont, I thought. I have to say, that as horrible as the accident had been, I welcomed the calm atmosphere of this little hospital relative to big city hospitals with all of their scary sights, sounds and smells. I didn't have to witness mangled faces and people walking around with IV poles, while I waited for care. I also marveled at, and would not soon forget, the soothing and wonderful manner of Charlene, the EMT. There were definitely advantages to small town life.

After examining me all over, the doctor declared that I suffered from shock but would otherwise survive, and that I should expect a couple of weeks of extreme soreness and nasty bruises. "In fact," the doctor stated, "for the next couple of days, it actually might be hard to turn your head back and forth. When you're in an accident, you end up tensing up and stressing muscles that you didn't even know you had. But otherwise, just take it easy and let me know if things don't start feeling better in a couple of weeks. Other than that, you're okay to go home. Just make sure someone else drives."

"Well, I don't think I have a car anymore, so that rule shouldn't be too hard to follow," I said, attempting to be droll. She made a sympathetic face at me and got ready to exit the makeshift room, probably to attend Pig Man (I heard his deep voice down the hall and upgraded him from "boy").

"Wait!" I said, desperation tingeing my voice. "I don't actually know anybody's phone numbers." I felt horribly embarrassed just saying these words. Could someone just find a "loser" stamp to decorate my forehead?

"You don't know anybody's phone number?" the doctor repeated in amused disbelief, or maybe that was concern. Perhaps I had a serious head injury, after all.

"I live in an inn that is shared by fifteen people and I don't ever call any of them because I can just walk to their rooms. I guess I could try to call the pub that's attached to the building and see if they can go upstairs and try to find somebody to come get me. This is crazy, because of course everyone's in class, where I should be right now, and half the people who live there don't even have cars." I was beginning to babble and could feel tears welling up in my eyes. Damn waterworks.

"All right, just give me a minute and I'll see what I can do." The doctor walked out. A half hour later, a nurse came in and said that a couple of people from my school had arrived to pick me up. When I reached the lobby, I was elated, and quite surprised, to see Jasper and Lanie, two students who each had rooms down the hall from me. They were waiting with worried expressions. I'd never felt so relieved to see friendly, familiar faces. They escorted me home, listened to the details about the crazy incident, spinning car, pig and all, and helped me negotiate the stairs up to my room. Still no word about my car, so I had to call. The police told me it had been towed, and that it looked totaled. I no longer had my car. I was grateful to have my life.

I tucked myself into bed and tried to relax. I heard the other students, including Jason, return from their afternoon classes and realized that he had no idea what had happened to me. I listened as Jasper gave him the details down the hall and how Jason wouldn't let him finish before grabbing his keys to head to the hospital thinking I was still there, hurt. I started yelling from my bed so that he would hear me and not hastily leave. He heard me; I could hear his footsteps run toward my room.

"Oh my God, are you alright? Where does it hurt? What can I do?" He was breathless and had a manic look in his eyes.

I reached up and touched his face. "It's okay. I'm okay," I reassured him. "Just a little fender-bender that totaled the car, that's all." His eyes grew large like two shiny half-dollars. "But no, really, I'm fine and pretty lucky. If the man had hit just a split second earlier he would've probably gotten my door rather than the back seat door and then things might've been a little different." I smoothed my thumb along his cheek, calming him as much as myself. "But the man's fine and I'm fine. Just a little shaken up. And I feel pretty stupid getting in an accident literally feet from the police department." Jason laughed at this and visibly relaxed.

"I tell you what, baby, I'm going to go run a quick errand and then I'll be back and we can just relax and watch movies and just take it easy, okay?" I smiled up at him and he kissed me gently on the forehead. He came back shortly thereafter with a gallon of my favorite ice cream, mint chocolate chip, and a couple of my favorite Audrey Hepburn movies. I realized, right then, if not a hundred times before, that I never wanted to lose him.

Later that night, I dialed the number to my father's hospital room and breathed with relief when he answered the phone. He sounded alert and awake; an excellent sign. I could hear him eating and decided I'd wait until a much later time to tell him about the accident, maybe months. How about a year? He just came out of surgery. I didn't want to throw him back in right away. We talked for a few minutes about hospital food and some pretty nurse, which I struggled to appreciate. Then he knocked the wind out of me.

"How's Puff?"

"What?" I asked, voice warbling in a nervous laugh. Did he have some kind of sixth sense? This wasn't the first time he'd asked just the right question.

"I haven't checked in on Puff in a while. How's Puff doing?"

"Well, funny you should ask. Puff and I had a little fender bender today."

"How bad?"

"She's gone, Dad. Puff is gone. I'm okay. In bed and a little bruised. But she's totaled." I heard him sigh.

"It's been a hell of a year, my dear." No shit, Dad. But, of course, I didn't say that out loud.

***

I had always heard that bad things come in threes, so I figured that between Mom's death, Dad's heart surgery and totaling my car, I'd covered the tragedy trifecta. Why, then, did I still live in fear every day? Why did my body protest and throw weird symptom after weirder symptom at me. The local doctor in town quickly grew to know me as I pleaded for appointments on at least a monthly basis. After the car wreck and handling my father's recovery issue, I threw myself into such a state of worry and general daily panic that my stomach hurt; sharp pains like an ice pick, or dull aches like a twisting of my abdominal muscles in a vice. I also had burning pain, as if I'd swallowed a breakfast of citrus and lighter fluid. I had centralized pain, specific pain, pain that wouldn't go away. I just knew I had cancer. The doctor sent me to the hospital to have a test done called a barium swallow, wherein I drank two jugs of thick chalky white fluid (although it had more the texture of loose paste), then reclined on a bed in a dark, terrifying room while they scanned by midsection every which way. Surprise! No cancer. The doctor suggested I try yoga or medication, or psychotherapy; anything to decrease stress.

Next, the ear fluttering materialized. For a month, my ear sounded as if a moth was trapped inside and continued to rapidly vibrate its wings to escape. I could hear fine, but everything had the added bonus of flapping on top of it. The moth made it extremely difficult to fall asleep, pay attention to anything, or simply exist. The doctor told me the Eustachian tubes in my ears were small, so if I had any cold or sinus issues, it was probably just a little fluid back-up. I wanted to marry the day that the ear fluttering finally subsided. I was certain that a large tumor had been pressing upon my ear drum.

"Are you sure it's not the altitude or something that's doing it?" I asked. The doctor almost fell off his stool, trying to contain his mirth.

"We're not really high right here. In fact we're in a valley and the mountains around us aren't even really high enough to cause any noticeable ear problems." I just know he wrote something about me in my chart after that.

Then, my eye started twitching. It randomly contorted for another, separate, whole month. I fought embarrassment daily as I tried to converse with professors, friends, vendors, small animals. They all looked at me as they talked, kind of cocking their heads to the side, wondering why one eye looked lazier than the other and kept sort of winking at them. I rushed to the doctor, sure of a stroke or some other type of palsy. The doctor sat me down and looked me in the eye and said, "You are too stressed out. You need to calm down." He patted me on my shoulder and I paid my co-pay (again) and left, tail between my legs. The twitching eventually stopped. Maybe all the madness would cease.

I had made it through a week or so with no strange bodily happenings. Jason and I ventured over to Hanover to take in an interesting lecture and movie about Frank Lloyd Wright at Dartmouth. These forays always kept me feeling academic and slightly superior; although I'm not really sure to whom. As we walked into the theater, we passed a little toddler wearing a tie-dyed jumper, his long dirty curls bouncing around his rosy cherub cheeks. He was completely barefoot.

"Wow," Jason said. "I never notice kids, but that's the cutest kid I've ever seen." This didn't surprise me considering that he went to a hippy undergrad school that chanted things like "let's all live together and love each other." He then said, "That's the kind of kid I want one day." My heart skipped about ten beats in a row, causing the icky light-headedness. I clumsily tripped over to the nearest water fountain to tame my wild heart rate. Did he just bring up having kids with me? The mere thought of having kids, the physical act of having kids, sent me into a spiral of vertigo. On a theoretical level, I, of course, wanted children. Two, maybe three. How I would manage the physical nature of actually having them, well, I didn't feel remotely ready to address that little problem.

"Can we go in and sit down?" I asked. I hoped I exuded calmness outwardly. I relaxed as I sat there, allowing all displaced blood to fill in the proper nooks and crannies of my body. The lights went out and within five minutes a hard and swift pulsing commenced in my stomach near my ribcage. It felt like the moth in my ear had grown into a giant creature and relocated south. A pattern developed and kept thumping away in my stomach. I had to leave the room after a while because I couldn't just sit there in the dark and do nothing. I ended up pacing back and forth outside the theater, plotting my next move. Should I head to the ER? Would I even make it there in time? Does Jason even know I'm gone? At intermission, he came out to find me.

"Where've you been? I thought you just went to the bathroom." I was helpless. I had to tell him, as sad as it would make him.

"Something's wrong," I said.

"Okay." He had learned not to overreact to my issues, as he rightly believed it would feed my anxiety. Instead he always waited patiently for me to explain before digesting the information and deciding how to respond. He was very wise.

"My stomach's fluttering. And it won't stop." I sounded alarmed. He looked at me, amused.

"You're fine. Just a muscle spasm. Now come on in and sit down. The movie's really good."

"You think?"

"I know."

"But you're not a doctor." I have used this line a lot. If he's in the right mood, he'll say, "But I'm almost a jurisdoctor." On really good days, he'll say, "I'm a doctor of love." Today he wasn't in the right mood.

"Just trust me, you'll be fine."

I made it through the rest of the movie and presentation and it eventually went away, after four days. I lost a lot of sleep during those days. But instead of going back to the doctor, I looked myself in the mirror and said, "You're too stressed. You need to relax."

Hypochondriac Lesson #14:
Take a vacation!

## *14- Escape to the Aegean*

"Aren't you Greek?" Well, considering this is the first thing I've heard that I understand, I should say, no, I am not Greek. I shook my head no, said "Sorry," shrugged my shoulders and smiled. The old woman continued rapidly in her tongue, ignoring the fact that I had no idea what she said. I listened politely. I had arrived in Greece, in Athens, only a couple of hours ago and sat waiting for my small plane to fly me to the island of Rhodos. This woman, covered from head to toe in a black, hooded frock, was actually the second person to assume my nationality as local. Maybe my thick eyebrows and dark hair confused them. Maybe I needed to tend to my pesky moustache. I would have thought my skin too fair to qualify as Mediterranean but I was new to this part of the world. What did I know? Hey, at least I fit in with the natives. For my first big travel adventure on my own, I considered my blending a blessing.

For two months, at the age of twenty-three, I had the pleasure of studying in the Greek Isles- Rhodos, the sensationally beautiful tiny island of Spetses, and Crete- as part of my law school curriculum. My classrooms overlooked the beach; the ocean a color so blue it seemed artificially enhanced by 1960's Technicolor. I spent days sunning myself by the pool, developing my first real tan, ever, and shopping along cobblestoned streets lined with white-washed buildings and magenta bougainvillea. Honestly, to call that summer "studying abroad" was almost comical. The addition of Supreme Court Justice Ruth Bader Ginsberg added the most distinctive hint that I participated in anything academic. I took the courses pass/fail. It was not a bad deal, overall. But me being, well, me, I encountered a few mental bumps in the road; even in paradise. Jason had proposed to me only a month before, and we would now live separately for the whole summer. I found my emotions in quite a pickle.

Over the last six months, I had developed what I termed "heart jumpies" and fell victim to these little attacks with increasing frequency. I would stand up fast, get nervous about something, or just sit and enjoy a TV show and all of a sudden my heart would leap out of control, skipping beats, mimicking the sensation of a little butterfly fluttering in my chest. The initial feeling would last less than a minute but my head would wrap around the memory of it like a pretty ribbon with a double knot. I fretted, feared and generally wouldn't let go of what had happened. I would go to sleep that night and worry nonstop that I would experience the same heart jumpies the next day and day after that. The minute I woke up heart jumpies jumped into my thoughts. If I could've beaten them out with a bat, I would have done so in an instant. Then I would worry about a head injury.

I stood up at the airport to say my tearful, choking goodbyes to Jason and a rousing bout of heart jumpies commenced. I dwelled on them, considering the finer nuances of their essences on the ten hour plane ride to Athens. Nervous about making my connecting flight to Rhodos and apprehension about navigating by myself around a foreign land sparked another round of the little bastards. They came like applause for each move I made; the anti-reward for making progress on my trip, or in my life for that matter. Once I landed in Rhodos, I knew I would need to find a cab and hope the driver spoke English so that I could make it to my hotel. Already late for the introductory meeting, I rushed into the airport bathroom to splash water in my face in order to quell the damn jumpies and my impending sick stomach brought on by a pounding transatlantic headache. A bottle of water would have gone a long way at this point.

Once I arrived, and checked into my hotel (so far, and much to my relief, everyone spoke English with Greek greetings sprinkled in like holiday confetti, which sort of made me disappointed in myself for wanting it to be that way), I found my way down to the conference room for the trip meeting. I instantly felt better once I saw the crowd of students my age and a row of professors at the head of the room. Okay, I can relax. It's all going to be okay. And there's a hospital only a mile away, in case it isn't okay. I'd checked to see my location in relation to a hospital. I wanted to know that if my jumpies lasted too long, I would have time to make it to the emergency room before I died. Do you think I might've had just a smidge of Post Traumatic Stress Disorder as a residual effect of watching my mother die? Once again, I was textbook; comforting and annoying at the same time. I could relax in this room now and hear about the next two months. Two months? When I signed up for this Study Abroad program, it sounded so awesome on paper. But now, sitting here with all of these strangers, a world away from my fiancé and my American doctors, I suddenly wondered if I'd gone mad by committing myself to such a long time away, at such a great distance. When I got back to my room, I phoned my father right away.

"What am I doing here?" He started laughing when he heard my voice.

"Not having fun, yet?" I could hear the grin in his voice.

"I feel like I'm going to be sick. How am I ever going to make it through these two months? That seems like a lifetime from now."

"Don't be ridiculous, Kat. You used to spend that amount of time at summer camp and not think anything of it."

"Yeah, well missing you guys just wasn't the same, I guess."

"Oh, you're missing your man, already? I see. You want me to make you feel better about missing Jason."

"That would be awfully kind of you."

"Okay. Here goes. Get a grip. You're in the Greek Isles for the summer. You're going to have the experience of a lifetime. Jason loves you and will be waiting anxiously for you when you get home. And he'll enjoy all of the detailed letters that you write him."

"Yeah, I guess you're right." I said, sighing.

"You're damn right, I'm right. Oh, poor Kat. Stuck on a beautiful island in Greece. Can you hear my violin?"

"Fine. I get it."

"You've just had long flights and you're tired. Get some sleep and enjoy this experience. It'll be good for you."

"Thanks, Dad." After I hung up, I felt better. I knew he was right and just hearing a familiar voice made me feel more grounded and not like I had entered another world entirely.

The next day I woke up to a cloudless blue sky. It would stay that way for the entire two months. I only saw one cloud the whole summer, alien in its attempt to live in the sky, putting a damper on perfection. I walked out onto the balcony, and stood there in awe. I hadn't noticed the balcony last night in my hazy stupor of dumping my bag. It would have been more bags, but the airlines lost my luggage, which added to my general indigestion upon arrival. I leaned on the rail, viewing the ridiculous gemstone azure hue of the water, and saw all the way to Turkey. I don't ever want to leave here. This is amazing. Too bad I had to wear the same outfit I wore yesterday, a dress stinky with travel and slight whiff of public bathroom. A small stain of airplane salad dressing adorned the front part of my dress that had been scrunched up in my lap as I ate in flight. I had already called the airline three times about my luggage and they informed me that they "might know something more soon. Call back in an hour." I detected they might be stalling. With a view like this, I guess I could survive a few more hours in old, dank clothes. I just had to make it through my one class for the day without putting people off with my appearance and stench. I arrived on a Sunday. By Tuesday, I assumed my suitcases had found a final resting place at the bottom of the ocean.

Unable to tolerate the looks from the other students (I didn't want to lose friends here), I had to cash some traveler's checks and give in to purchasing one or two outfits to see me through until my clothes finally appeared. I walked out after class and ventured down the street to find something to wear. I'm not quite sure how it happened, if maybe I had a stroke along the way, but instead of a couple of suitable outfits for class I ended up with a new bikini, strapless cover-up and skimpy spaghetti strap dress in both solid black and spicy floral pattern. Well, then. When in the Greek Isles...

I've always loved traveling. We only took cruises when I was young, as my mother feared flying to such a degree that we needed to provide her with a paper bag to simply discuss the topic. I cruised all over the Caribbean and Mexico. Living in Florida, we had easy access to the ports. We also took a fair amount of road trips to visit friends, but never anything north of the Carolinas. I ached for far reaching travel from as early as I can remember. I devoured travel guides and brochures at the agencies where my parents booked cruises; well before the prevailing online bookings. I read all about the European countries in our 1952 set of World Book Encyclopedias. The World Showcase of Epcot Center became my very own fantasy land. I have photos of me wearing a beret in "France" and a striped shirt in "Italy." Did I think I was a gondolier? I shook my Maracas in "Mexico;" not as sexual as it sounds; and tried to make a beefeater laugh at the "United Kingdom." My parents recognized my wanderlust and upon graduation, sold an antique silver punch set to afford to send me to Europe on a six country tour for the summer. I never looked back and the travel bug only grew and nibbled at my brain. Unable to afford the extra expenses in college to study abroad, I swore to myself I would take care of business in law school. Voila, I wound up in Greece for a summer.

I decided to take advantage of every opportunity. The group leaders and teachers would post excursion and travel opportunities for our weekends and afternoons and I signed up for every single one, not caring about the details. The other students made fun of me, calling me lame for having such a gung ho attitude towards excursions. As Flo from "Alice" would say, "Kiss my grits." Wasn't I here to see Greece? I planned to see as much as possible. I could sit on the beach back in the States. I immediately signed up for the trip to a small island on Saturday and sailing on Sunday.

On Saturday, our boat, the size of a medium fishing boat, ferried about fifteen of us to a tiny island with a population of less than two hundred people. With one church and one restaurant and stunning views, it felt like we'd discovered a mini utopia. At lunch, the food tasted so delicious and authentic. We ate large bricks of feta with slices of watermelon, the sweet and salty complimenting each other in a glorious burst of flavor. We polished off beans the size of a baby's fist, floating in olive oil and red sauce, and savored the divine texture of the grape leaves stuffed with rice. I didn't want to stop eating. The Mediterranean diet is good for you, right? We concluded the meal with a shot of ouzo, typical of most Greek meals, a surprisingly satisfying digestive. We visited the church, hiked up the small hill to some old ruins, then reclined on the beach to enjoy the slow pace of life and gorgeous scenery. What a beautiful day.

The next day, I woke up and threw up. And kept throwing up. I threw up until I thought I might die, throwing up. I have never experienced this duration or violence of sickness. My poor roommate called at me from outside the bathroom door. I know she obviously needed to use it at some point that morning, but I couldn't physically leave it. Not for a second. I sat by the toilet, unable to move, limbs so heavy they felt like stones from the previous day's acropolis had decided to stow away and make an escape from the little island. I'd stripped all my clothes off so that I wouldn't ruin anything. I still hadn't received my luggage after a week and couldn't afford to keep buying clothes. Could I wear a bikini to class? Perhaps the feta did this to me; a difference in the whole pasteurization process, maybe? Oh, don't talk about the feta. Don't even mention anything that I ate. I called the trip leader and cancelled my trip on the sailboat for the day. The mere thought of the swaying and bouncing over the seas in my condition pushed me further into porcelain. I called a new acquaintance to beg her to get me some lemon Fanta, the closest thing to a 7up or Ginger Ale I could think of, from the hotel sundries store. I could not even keep the smallest sip of water down. I started to shake and felt so tired and weak. My heart rate would not slow down. The fear crept up on me. Would I have to go to a foreign hospital? Would they be able to help me? I called the trip leader back and pleaded for help. She called a doctor and convinced one to make a house call to me in my hotel room. An hour later, a short Greek man with dark hair, dark tanned skin and dark brown eyes entered my room and told me to lie down flat in my bed.

"Hmm," he said, while pushing around on my stomach. Um, you might not want to do that, as I've been creating my own little fountain of antiquity here this morning.

"What's hmm?" I asked. He looked at me perplexed. He didn't understand why I had questions yet, didn't understand the hypochondriac.

"You have traveler's stomach." He said it matter-of-factly, no need for questions or discussion. "Did you have any vegetables yesterday?"

"Yes, I had the large white beans."

"Yes, people are always worried that the meat will be what makes them sick. But no, it's usually the vegetables, because of how they are washed and treated. It's different than what your stomach is used to."

"I see. Any idea of when I'll get better? This is awful."

"Couple of days. Eat only rice. White rice. And yogurt. Only real Greek yogurt. This is the only kind that will help you." If I didn't know better, I would think he received a commission from the Greek Yogurt people, he was so adamant.

The following day or two, I imposed on the kindness of strangers to fetch me yogurt (easy, it's everywhere) and white rice (not so easy to find, because even in the numerous Chinese restaurants, the rice is covered in oil). In the meantime, I watched Tennis championships, fixated on Andre Agassi without the long hair, on TV in my room and marveled at Greek commercials. Can you guess what three naked people playing with each other's hair sells? Drum roll. Orange juice. I could never figure out the advertising in this country. Then JFK Junior's plane went down. Then Egypt Air crashed a plane. At that point I started having a few dehydration induced panic attacks. I was already nervous about all the flying and ferrying and traveling awaiting me. While I loved to visit destinations, the actual transportation part always made me a twittering wreck. I called Jason and my father quite a few times after hearing of these tragedies; plastered all over the Greek news non-stop. Even in another language, they were catastrophic and horrible. If I was to share the same fate and only had a short time left among the living to express my love, I needed them to know. I ended up owing more on my credit card for phone calls at the end of the summer than all my other souvenir, travel and food expenses combined. Oops. When I could stand moving my body again, I ventured out onto the balcony and basked in sunlight and serenity, and a view of the mini golf course on the property, while I wrote things like "Lord, please help me to stop being so crazy" and "I want to feel better; why can't I stop having dizzy spells" and "I keep having cravings for orange juice" in my daily diary.

Eventually the dense Greek yogurt and the white rice, oily as it came, did the trick and I recovered. I managed to regain full regard for all the food available, aside from the baby fist white beans. I thought it best to avoid tempting fate; mythology was big around these parts. At my next healthy opportunity, I decided to set off exploring. I took a ferry to the island of Symi one Saturday, a lovely little island with the town perched on the side of its steep topography. I lost myself and track of time meandering through the narrow streets and alleys, winding higher until I discovered I had reached the top, literally, of town and looked down at the whole of its buildings and structures with the sea serving as an impressive backdrop. This was beautiful; a feast for the senses. I sat down, rested, and realized that I had not thought about my heart rate or dizziness all day. Until then, of course, from which time I struggled to think about anything else. But I congratulated myself for forgetting my idiocy for at least a little while. I walked back down the steep stairs and paths and browsed the little shops, then stopped into a restaurant to dine on some fresh prawns sprinkled with my beloved feta, hoping the cholesterol wouldn't kill me. Food doesn't work the same negative effects on your body while you travel, right? That's only the day-to-day dining that clogs the arteries. That's my theory, and for these purposes, I'm sticking to it.

At some point, I glanced at my watch, more out of curiosity than necessity, and then sat still, looking at the numbers before my eyes. That can't be right. It can't be almost seven. The last ferry leaves at six. Wait, am I reading this wrong? Realization dawned on me like a new morning. I couldn't be that dumb. Oh, crap. I've missed my ferry. I slowly paid the waitress, picked up my bag and darted for the dock. Please, please, please still be there. For my sake, be late like every other time I want to get somewhere. No such luck. The last ferry had indeed left. Fifteen minutes ago. So what would a single American girl like me do now? I had no cell phone. I didn't have much money, couldn't really afford a hotel. Guess I shouldn't have bought that bikini. I had a perfectly good bathing suit already. As I chastised myself, I could feel the tears stinging my eyes. I must have appeared quite the sight; floppy blue hat to protect me from the vicious sun, pink tank top, khaki shorts, backpack/purse hybrid with inside zipper that snuggled up against the body so thieves would have a harder time mugging me, slooped shoulders, and wet face. I smelled of sunscreen and American tourist. I might as well have had a fanny pack. I passed by a woman closing up her shop for the day, pulling in her clothes racks and wrought iron mannequins.

"Hey, are you okay?" she asked, clearly concerned. I noticed her English was very good.

"Oh, I'll be fine. I just missed the last ferry back to Rhodos and now I don't know what to do." I started crying at this point, full force. She dropped the bin she carried and ran over to me, wrapping her arms around me in a giant hug. The action completely caught me off guard and I stopped crying immediately, replaced with the sudden urge to laugh.

"I tell you what. You'll stay with me and my family. You are American, no?" I nodded my head yes, but nervously. I'd seen the posters in Athens of Bill Clinton's head on the body of Godzilla and wasn't sure where everyone stood with American politics and views about Americans overall. "We have plenty of room and I will make you something good, like spaghetti that you are probably missing from home. Then tomorrow morning, I'll bring you down to the ferry and make sure you get back to Rhodos. Tonight you are part of our family." This was why I would always want to travel.


After my stint in Rhodos, the program moved to the tiny lovely island of Spetses. The entire diameter of the island did not exceed five miles or so, but the place oozed with charm, a little bit of magic and a lot of yachts. By this point in the summer, the temperature gauge started rising. Without a cloud to provide any shade or relief, the days developed a kind of sizzle. Each day, I would walk from our beach front hotel into town to the shops and restaurants. I started carrying one of those nerdy little water bottles with a fan attached that would blow and spray at the same time. While mildly satisfying, it did not solve the problem of the direct sunlight on my head, cooking my brains like a campfire foil dinner. Was the big-haired girl with the mini fan attractive? Not so much, but I had to take the prudent course given my history with heat exhaustion.

One afternoon, while walking in the arid heat of about 101 degrees, I felt myself lose it. My stomach churned and flipped about. My heart twitched into jumpies mode and my head spun. My vision starting blurring around the edges and I could feel my face flush hotter than the sun. Just as my body commenced falling towards the ground and heaviness overcame me, I heard a rumbling noise in the distance. Yanni, or Stelios-everyone was named one of these, it seemed- an employee of my hotel; who I later heard through rumors had slept with three different students from my trip; pulled up next to me on his scooter, and said, "Vroom, vroom." He did not rev the engine of the scooter, but actually said the words, "Vroom, vroom." Temporarily pulled out of my about-faint by the ludicracy of his words, I managed to say, "What?"

"You want a ride?" He raised his eyebrows up and down, quickly. Was he hitting on me? Maybe I appeared to be swooning over his swarthiness and scooterificness. Either way, I didn't care. He could be my hairy savior. I hopped on the back of that thing so fast Yanni didn't even have time to continue with his witty repartee. I just needed to find air conditioning and a horizontal position. And no, not with Yanni. He did seem a little disappointed when I hopped off and ran to my room alone when we got back to the hotel. Who cares? Thank goodness for horny men on scooters.

I continued to struggle with the heat and heart jumpies throughout the trip, but managed to always find a safe place where the jumpies would stop and I could cool down. I did not, however, have the opportunity to escape my roommate and her episodes. I felt blessed that the trip leaders had placed me with Sandra for the portion of my studies in Spetses and Crete. She was funny, independent and mouthy. Easy to talk to, we hit it off right away and looked forward to an exciting seven weeks together. Then she started complaining about her back hurting. Then she started struggling to breathe. She'd never had such issues before and the episodes terrified her. Watching them take place, they certainly terrified me, too. She would double over and stay there, trying to make it pass. Only, I had no idea what she needed to pass. The trip leaders called the doctors, who diagnosed her with asthma. She had to carry around an inhaler from that point forward and ended up using it almost daily. So sudden, and so strong, the episodes made her feel a couple of times like she might die. As you can imagine, I FREAKED out. I was only two years out of my mother's death and the similarities of the back pain and difficulty breathing touched a little too close to home for me. I wanted to support Sandra as much as possible, but I had no idea how to help her or what I would do if something happening to her. I prayed a lot during that time.

I somehow lost touch with Sandra after the trip, so I have no idea about her final diagnosis once back in the States. I had much difficulty getting over the fact that such serious symptoms could flare up seemingly out of nowhere and so quickly. My sleeping hours held many nightmares after that.

\*\*\*

Perhaps you wonder why I share these little tales from my travels and studies in Greece. Well, this was the first time in years that I actually felt like I'd started to reclaim myself again. I'd made the voyage alone and had lived through amazing experiences that allowed me to feel like the strong, independent person I'd been before my mother died. Clearly, I still worried about a lot of issues, and would need to dedicate more time to working through those. But I found a little bit of myself in those ruins that had been missing for a while. When I negotiated the price down for my leather jacket and then ate apricots out of the store owner's garden, discussing life with him and his wife, I found that old debater in me again. When I hiked down the steep, creepy stairs deep into the dark cave considered to be Zeus's birthplace, I realized that my adventurous spirit did not exist only on hiking trails and pinnacles with Jason. When I snapped a picture with Justice Ginsberg, standing side-by-side with oversized sun hats and our donkeys in the background, I remembered that I have a cultivated sense of humor and exploratory nature. When I sat alone on the rooftop creperie in Spetses, owned by two friendly brothers, and ate Nutella crepes infused with ouzo, while staring at the insanely blue sea, I realized that even with all of my nuttiness, I do have an inner peace and serenity in there somewhere. It's just buried very deeply. For the first time, I felt like I was really giving time to me and that I could learn from all my fears. In order to conquer my fears, I needed to face them head-on and let the outcome work itself out. I now knew I was strong enough.

It's amazing the revelations you can make when faced with the opportunity of a clear perspective. Too bad every day isn't about thinking clearly.

Hypochondriac Lesson #15:
Eat right and exercise.

## *15- Is That A Wig, or Did I Drink Too Much?*

"Now just remember, you need to try to keep each other from gaining too much weight. Just because you're getting married, doesn't mean you can let yourselves go." My father-in-law-to-be bestowed this pearl of wisdom on us as he dropped us off at the Port of Miami, where we would embark on a seven day cruise to the Caribbean, courtesy of a winning raffle ticket at a recent wedding show for upcoming brides. We also needed to celebrate our hard-earned law degrees and take a little break from wedding plans and studying for the Bar Exam that summer. And now, apparently, go on a crash diet. My thinking about this statement was that he said it in innocence, not meaning to offend, but with an underlying message that Jason and I needed to think about our bodies a little more. Let's face the truth, we had gained weight. Too many pints of Ben and Jerry's factory seconds in Vermont; which often meant they'd included too MANY chunks of brownies or cookie dough; too much comfort food like shepherd's pie and not enough exercise. Sure, we hiked sometimes and skied a couple of times, but it's awfully cold in the winter, getting dark at four p.m., and mostly all you desire is curling up under a blanket with hot chocolate and food. Isn't that nature's way of helping you stay warm? It's what bears do. Frankly, though, I found his comment ill-timed. Nobody loses weight on a cruise, which offers twenty-four hours of food and a midnight buffet comprised entirely of chocolate. I've heard people brag about such a feat, but I've never seen the evidence, like a unicorn or some rare creature in the jungle that you have to sit quietly and wait for patiently for days, in hope of catching a glimpse, and if you're lucky, a photograph. From my previous cruising experiences, daintiness perished in a kind of warped survival of the fittest, or fattest, where gluttony rules the floating kingdom.

When my father-in-law said the words, I understand he did so with a pure heart and entirely free of malice. I looked down at myself instinctively. In my head, because I wouldn't speak of such ugliness out loud, I contemplated the size twelve pants I currently wore. Really, they had a cut that was more in line with a ten. Ahem. I'm trying to make myself feel better. Just go with me here. Needless to say, I'd never worn this size before. I am not terribly tall and my medium boned frame doesn't really support the weight very flatteringly. I had a hunch I'd fallen outside the healthy weight range for my body type. With parents who lived their entire adult lives overweight, Father-in-Law had a point. I needed to watch myself. I would even try my hardest on this cruise. In my mind, overweight people had heart disease, diabetes, and inevitably died young. I would not suffer the same fate. I promised myself to toss these ugly mint-colored size twelve pants- a minute ago I thought the color was SO Miami- as soon as we had the first opportunity to change. I didn't even need to have that number around. And who wears mint green pants anyway?

I couldn't wait for this cruise. I'd joined my parents on about eight or so from the age of eight to eighteen and always fantasized about wiling away the hours in the secluded little bars, crevices and niches of a ship with a sexy man all my own. As a girl, before a trip, I would try on all my new clothes purchased specifically for vacation, younger versions of resort wear, then toss my hair and talk to myself in the mirror, trying to come up with jazzy pick up lines and come hither looks. If I had to evaluate those moments, I would go with amateur and utterly embarrassing. But outside of my youthful quests for shipboard seduction on the high seas, I had so many fond memories. The moment that pops immediately to mind, actually forever branded into my mind, as if with a smoldering southwestern metal rod was when my father decided to partake in the passenger lip synch contest and

"sing" a fabulous rendition of "New York, New York." Without the aid of alcohol, he
waddled out onto the stage wearing a black top hat, black shoes (old man Velcro
style), black socks and a black diaper my mother had fashioned out of fabric. I
have no idea where she obtained this fabric; it is still a mystery. She had painted
"I <heart> NY" onto his rear end with red fabric paint. I'm not clear why he
decided on this get-up, or how it really pertained to the song. At that point, my
father was around fifty years old. Light brown hair covered his chest and belly, the
latter of which remained taut not with six pack abs, but as if he had swallowed a
basketball whole. His belly did not give when poked; just stayed firm. His skinny
arms and short scrawny legs seemed to orbit around his midsection and were
clearly in on the joke. Upon entering the stage, the audience fell silent in shock,
and then roared collectively in guffawing, disbelieving laughter. Women starting
throwing their room keys on stage, and at one point a hot pink bra grazed his
stomach as he swiveled and kicked past, lifting his top hat up and down in time to
the music. We were told by the Princess Cruise Line staff that the video recording
of the event was selling better than they had ever seen. As I walked by myself on
the Lido deck one afternoon, I passed a TV replaying the blessed event, pretending
I had no idea of the identity of that crazy man. That's the kind of behavior from a
parent that can really send a teenager over the edge. Ah, good times.

But back to my current love cruise. We boarded the ship and discovered
our "quaint" inside cabin; about ten square feet with bunk beds and no windows
or natural light. Charming, romantic, opulent? No, those words would not
describe this speck of a dark cave space. Free! Ah, yes, that's the magic word I
seek. Therefore, for two law school graduates with no money and a huge amount
of student loan debt entering repayment in a couple of months, the room was
perfect. As my father, the cruise aficionado, once elegantly put it, "It doesn't

matter what kind of cabin you have. You're never in there, except to bang." Still, we had won this from a wedding show. This room did not smack of beautiful romance, honeymoon style. But I had to give it to the contest officials, it was intimate.

We attempted to put our luggage into the room at the same time as our bodies, and said a little prayer against claustrophobia before heading up on deck to seek out our muster station for the mandatory safety drill. I don't care for the drill, as it reminds me that even on vacation, I might die a horrible drowning death. Although, with the "women and children first" bit for boarding life boats, I guess I have a decent chance at survival. I would never leave Jason on the doomed ship, though, waving tearfully at me as I row to safety and he anticipates his impending demise. See, my mind always goes to these scenes. We also went, of course, to find food. The first buffet had already started, before the ship even sailed away from port. Maybe just one pina colada for me, then. I mean, it's almost rude not to have an umbrella drink in hand for the festive send-off to sea.

That evening we sashayed, arm-in-arm, into the main dining room to meet our seating partners for the first time. We found ourselves at a table for eight, four different couples. Over the years, I have had all kinds of experiences sharing a table with strangers on cruises. On my first cruise, at age ten, my family shared the table with a family from Alberta, Canada who became wonderful friends of ours. Their daughter, my age, accompanied me to shipboard activities and we even entered the costume contest together and won dressed as babies. She actually owned the same random Disney t-shirt as me and we wore them as twins. Other times, I've sat with older couples who emit sweetness and kindness and are pleasant to dine with, but with whom I didn't have much in common. I have never had dining companions quite like the ones I proudly introduce now.

Couple number one, to our left: two women traveling together, clearly lesbians, but fighting this fact with every last drop of their beings; at least outwardly. One, Helen, had short blond Ellen hair, a pretty, unadorned face, blue eyes and a thin frame. She smiled a lot and seemed very sweet but didn't say much. Lisa, her roommate/companion/lover, had an olive complexion, course reddish/blondish/brownish hair, the result of a repeated and/or bad dye job, that still had residual effects of a long ago perm; some curl, but mostly frizz. Her stocky, solid build dwarfed Helen and put the rest of us on alert. Her eyes indicated that she might find a way to kick each of our asses by the end of the cruise. Lisa did not smile. Lisa scowled to show she was enjoying the trip. Lisa snapped at Helen all the time. I imagined the bickering stemmed from a denial of their true nature and love for each other. Maybe I was wrong. But for two people who spent the funds to take a cruise, they did not seem to enjoy each other's company and appeared entirely mismatched.

Couple number two, directly across the table from us: another pair of women. This pair blasted their excitement down the decks like a bullhorn. For the week, they had escaped the monotony of family life to enjoy a Girlfriend's Getaway. Shelley had blond hair, strongly resembled Blythe Danner in style, smile and haircut. She had four boys at home she talked about endlessly, and a husband she described simply as "into sports." Sweet and happy-go-lucky, Shelley was pleasant to talk to, share dinner with and hear about her day on the ship or at port. Cassandra, her travel companion, on the other hand, boasted, shrieked and otherwise made a scene on a nightly basis. With honey colored layered locks and a face masked with far too much makeup, in an ill advised attempt to disguise her age, Cassandra made a habit of saying rather inappropriate things, or pretty much whatever she had on her mind, at startling loud volumes. I found it interesting that Shelley would befriend such a creature, and like her to such a degree as to share a cabin with her for a whole week. We each have our own tastes, I guess.

Couple number three, to our right: Marissa and Bill. Marissa arrived at the table on the first night, long and lean, in a tight black dress, long platinum hair and tarted up makeup. She had already secured a tan all over her body; I can't be sure of the realness of said tan; but her face remained strangely pale, like she'd repeatedly forgotten the sunscreen everywhere else but her face. The effect made her appear as an apparition, on spring break from the afterworld. Bill sported a mullet of pure brown and grease and wore jeans and a bolo tie. While the pair didn't scream "class," they seemed to complement each other well. When Marissa sat down, Cassandra said, "Well, aren't you the Barbie Doll." Marissa turned her petite nose up at her, frowning, and accepted all the other introductions but hers, basically ignoring her and skipping over her in the conversation. Jason and I nudged each other under the table. This could get really interesting. Bill fondled Marissa throughout the meal; seriously did not stop touching her the entire time. He even ate one-handed. Marissa's meal only contained a small side salad. The waiter didn't seem to understand her request. Passengers typically chose a soup and/or salad, appetizer, entrée and dessert. He couldn't get a grasp that "small side salad" would be the whole meal. When he had turned away, dismayed and confused, I inquired if she found the menu not to her liking. "Oh, I'm not a big eater," she said. I see. What about breathing? Is that one of your hobbies? I enjoy my heart beating and urinating. I count them among my favorite past times. I also realized that I had found the metaphorical unicorn, the one person who came on a cruise and did not eat. Fascinating. I felt like digging out a magnifying class and lab coat to begin my studies of her. Cassandra, meanwhile, snorted at Marissa.

"Not a big eater, eh? Maybe you should think about it. Put a little meat on those bones." She laughed at herself. Nobody else laughed. I quietly took a sip of my water. Bill laughed light-heartedly and falsely.

"No, my girl's perfect just like she is. Right, baby?" He moved his hand from the small of her back up to the shoulder furthest from him and rubbed in a circle. She turned to him and Eskimo kissed him by rubbing noses then returning her gaze to the rest of us.

"That's right, Pookie." Okay, now I couldn't be sure that I would keep my meal down.

That night, Jason and I congratulated ourselves for our luck. We couldn't have asked for a more eccentric crew with which to dine. In fact, we could just sit back and enjoy the show. How divine! The next night, nobody showed up at dinner. Crap. That didn't last long. Jason and I sat at the large round table by ourselves wondering when our entertainment would all forgive each other and decide to break bread together again.

Meanwhile, we enjoyed the cruise. We ate, we drank, we gambled modestly; we didn't really have a lot of extra cash lying around to just throw away; we learned to ballroom dance, which was super handy for our upcoming nuptials, we took a Catamaran through St. John's, we took afternoon tea accompanied by music from a grand piano (so posh), and enjoyed each other's company (wink, wink) in our "cozy" little cabin. The ship got a bit rocky one night and I fell out of the bottom bunk we had been attempting to share. I incurred a little hip bruise, but I claimed it came from a ballroom dancing lift; we were such fast learners; a regular Fred and Ginger. Then we ate some more.

The night of the Captain's Ball arrived and we dolled ourselves up to meet the captain and obtain the free drinks in his honor before dinner. I put on my black, off-the-shoulder, Vera Wang I had worn in a wedding two years before. Yes, I had managed to find a way to re-wear a brides maid dress. Jason zipped me up and

I stood there facing the mirror, turning puce. This used to zip right up and rest

comfortable on my body. It had allowed me to dance the night away in a country

club somewhere in Atlanta. Now, I could not breathe. Did the drycleaners shrink

this thing? Oh my god, I'm really getting fat. This hurt to realize, both emotionally

and, well, physically. I could see the zipper aching and straining, the teethed lines

desperately clinging to each other, but having difficulty staying attached to the

fabric at the same time; a veritable tug-o-war. Only, I would be the only loser, in

a torn dress. I dug out the control-top pantyhose that I brought, which I hate, but

now found essential to wear. Good. If I held my breath for most of the night, this

just might work. I started to sweat. That's glamorous.

We stiffly stood in line to have our portraits taken. Nothing says beauty like

holding your breath and grimacing. We stiffly walked by the captain to shake his

hand in his receiving line, then even more stiffly journeyed to the other end of

the ship for dinner. I had downed only half a glass of champagne as I didn't think

I would be able to add any volume to my body without the dress exploding off

of me in release. I took short little breaths and hoped that supplied my blood and

lungs with enough oxygen, but I figured it didn't since I started to notice a little

light-headedness. I felt like Scarlett O'Hara after the women help tie her into her

dress, cinching her into confinement, only without the sixteen inch waist. I will

not disclose my waist size; are you kidding? We finally completed this nonsensical

charade of high society and made it to our table. Much to our surprise the rest

of the table sat there, as if waiting patiently just for us before starting a greatly

anticipated reunion dinner.

"Well, lookie here. Don't you guys look like Kennedys? I didn't realize we had

American Royalty right at our table," said a woman with dark brown hair. Wait,

is that Cassandra? Is that a wig? Her hair looked like a pair of ferrets had decided to mate while on her head, with bends and swirls jutting out in all directions like tails. I expected to see it move any minute, like the slime that John Cusack's bad cook mother prepares in "Better Off Dead." Just pretend like everything is normal. She looked strange and I suddenly started to fear that she had cancer. But I actually think the wigs were her attempt at fashion diversity, a way to change things up and make her life more unpredictable and exciting. Maybe she wanted to test to see if blondes or brunettes really do have more fun. I laughed nervously at her comments; although as usual, nobody else responded to her at all, not even her travel partner; and hoped to the Almighty that they wouldn't hear the threads break as I attempted to sit down. I sort of leaned way back, while keeping my back straight so that I didn't entirely bend at the waist. I did not look comfortable, I can tell you that, and I didn't even have a view of myself. I pretended I had a board behind me but at a forty-five degree angle. The satin still cut into my stomach at a sharp angle at the pull line across my midsection, like a pretty, shiny blade. I would have paid a million dollars to have a sweater I could put on, so that I could unzip the back, just a hair, and allow myself the smidge of breathing room, undetected, that my body fervently craved. Oh no! I'm going to have to start wearing elastic all the time, like those people at buffet restaurants who wear the clothes that can grow with them and their meals. Oh horror! I will be forever destined to sweatpants and elder polyester.

I fought through the pain of the digging abdominal fold of the dress to eat some escargot; my favorite, and only served on fancy night; I refused to miss it. I indulged in some surf and turf, and baked Alaska. Come on, I couldn't miss that! Marissa decided to go with chilled cucumber soup as her meal, but declared it too heavy and filling to finish. Bill stroked her back, and I daresay, her butt cleavage throughout the meal. Shelley showed off her new jewelry purchase, a necklace composed of small diamond encrusted starfish that "my husband will kill me for, but Cassandra insisted I get." Cassandra snorted, with a detectable touch of evil. Helen sat serenely next to Lisa, who I almost didn't recognize due to the startling level of baking she had endured during the interim days. The pair admitted they had done not much of anything besides lay out; and tried to admit their true feelings for each other is my guess. Helen apparently opted for sun screen, while Lisa must have slathered on bacon grease and held a tin foil shield up to her face. She looked scary dark, like I wanted to hand her the card for my dermatologist, kind of dark.

"So, I see you haven't developed a taste for eating, yet," said Cassandra, winningly, to Marissa. Marissa just rolled her eyes and smiled at her Pookie, like an inside joke just passed between them. Again, nobody responded. I hated to miss the next oddity, but my discomfort had gone from worse to worst.

I excused myself, told Jason I needed to head back to the cabin, and scurried out of the dining room as fast as my short breaths would carry me; not very fast, in case you were wondering. As I reached behind to unzip my dress, contorting like a soft, doughy hot pretzel sweating salt, I felt the relief waft through my organs with each inch the zipper traveled south. Ah, I could finally take a whole, cleansing, fulfilling breath. I took the dress off and laid it on the bed in front of me. I looked at it curiously, like I might an alien or a foreign artifact. I searched for a reason why a simple black dress that I had once worn and loved could have turned on me so viciously. But I knew I could really only blame myself. What had I done to myself? I knew better than this. I should have already learned my lesson. Didn't I have the family proof necessary to make the right decisions about my health? Clearly the Munster cheese on bagels for breakfast would not help matters, or the cheesecake we had eaten to celebrate graduation, or any of the mess of food on this cruise. I needed air. I changed into a loose sundress and left Jason a note.

I slowly walked around the ship, unsure of any real destination. I strolled aimlessly, passing by lovers walking hand-in-hand and children excitedly circling their parents, telling them all about the scavenger hunt they had done that afternoon. I found myself on an outside deck with open railings and decided to stand for a while, overlooking the moon and its reflection upon the inky black water. Wow, I was living a Love Boat episode. Maybe Doc or Gopher would come out and try to make me feel better while Isaac poured me a drink from any bar I happened to pass. That guy was everywhere. Then it hit me. After almost three years since my mother had passed away, this was my first visit to her final resting place. I had always had trouble dealing with the fact that they scattered her ashes at sea and I had no place to visit to mourn properly. But now, here I stood; officially "At Sea." Believe me; I understand that the small quantity of her ashes did not occupy the whole sea. But they were in here somewhere and her spirit, I had learned, hovered everywhere. This was as good as I was going to get.

"Hello Mommy," I said, looking around to make sure nobody walked by and saw me talking to myself.

"It's good to be here." Let's see, what do I say? "I miss you." That was certainly the truth. "I'm here with my fiancé. Have you seen him? He's really cute and nice. I think he's the one and I wish you could meet him. I think you'd like him."

I paused and looked down at my hands. They had started to fiddle with each other as I leaned on the rail.

"I'm not sure what to say. Dad and Katrina are doing okay. I think they'd be better with you here. But I understand that you can't be here in person. Finally. It took me a while to make that stick. You were far too young to go. Did you want to leave?" I looked up into the sky as if I might hear a response from somewhere.

People talked to the dead and discussed it on talk shows all the time. "Well, your timing was bad for us. Although probably better for you, given Dad's heart attack. You probably wouldn't have enjoyed that too much. I already know you couldn't handle the no money thing. But," and here's where I started getting teary, "you're going to miss my wedding. I wish so much that you could've been here to help me plan it. I went to my shower last week before this trip and it just wasn't the same without you. You should have been there. And you should've helped me pick out my dress and helped me decide what to do with my hair. And I should've been able to help you pick out a nice dress or suit for the Mother of the Bride." I paused. I truly believed she already knew all of this. She watched all the events of my life and my sister's life. I didn't need to fill her in. But I could tell her how I felt.

"Why couldn't you just get some help? I know you were depressed. Why couldn't you take medicine? I know you and Dad had lost a lot, but we could've all worked together to make it better. It didn't have to be the end. You could have taken better care of yourself." I inwardly chastised myself for scolding the dead. No use dragging up old problems. What was done was done.

"Well, now I'm getting married and I'm fat. It's like I haven't learned anything from you at all. I don't want to die when I'm forty-four. I don't want to have low self esteem about my body. I want to be healthy and thin and happy." I stared out into the water for a long time in silence. "I really miss you, Mommy. God, I wish you could come back to us."

A week later, after the cruise, the gorge-fest of indulgences, I went to the doctor for my annual physical and asked her to check my cholesterol and blood sugar. I got the call a few days later.

"Kat, your triglycerides are a little elevated and while your overall cholesterol is in the normal range, your good cholesterol needs to be higher and your bad cholesterol needs to be lower," the doctor said, as my mind started hearing static. She continued to talk and I'm sure it was very important, but all I could hear in my mind was, "You are going to die, just like your mother."

Hypochondriac Lesson #16:
Sometimes crap happens (pun intended)
and you just have to deal with it.

*16- Get Hitched and Hurl*

"To Kat and Jason, and a long happy life together," said my father, the toaster. This simple statement ended a speech that had brought him to choking tears, stumbling jelly legs, and an utterance about his wife being gone. It was sweet, melancholy and almost too much to bear.

"Here, here," everyone replied, lifting their glasses. Sensing a reprieve in the speeches, I leaned over and whispered into Jason's ear.

"I'm going to head out now to the bathroom and take a Tums." He looked at me, not so much with concern, he was getting used to me by now, but with amusement.

"How many rolls did you bring? We still have a couple of hours left. We've only had the salads." He smiled.

"Very funny. I won't be long." I kissed him and darted furtively out of the room, as if people wouldn't notice that the bride-to-be had exited the Rehearsal Dinner. I just didn't want to throw up in front of them. I had no qualms about marrying Jason, no cold feet; in fact they felt almost too warm in these heels. I just didn't want the heart jumpies to keep me from walking down the aisle properly. I didn't want to collapse at the altar, and I kept having visions of passing out and everyone gasping and clustering around me as I perished on the floor trying to revive my large satiny self. I had already devoured two rolls of Tums thinking about the possibilities. I had not touched my salad and once I saw the waiters start to walk in with the almond encrusted haddock, the churning told me I would not eat any of that either. I entered the bathroom and stared at myself hard and scoldingly in the mirror. Pull yourself together, Kat. You're just getting married. If anything, there will be plenty of people who can call 911 if you have a heart attack. You're just having nerves. I dabbed some cold water on the back of my neck from the faucet. I would have splashed it in my face, but thought that returning to the dining room with a wet face and running mascara might give my insanity away. Might as well let people continue with the illusion that I was poised and calm. I straightened my pearls, returning the clasp to the back, dried myself off, smoothed my simple black dress and also the loose wisps of hair in my chignon, and adjusted my posture to walk back out to the group with an Audrey Hepburn air of confidence. I still couldn't eat that darn fish. I took another Tums.

My wedding day dawned the next day with a perfectly clear Florida sky. August in Orlando; hot as a fry cooker and quite humid, but so far, so good on the blue sky. I had left Jason after the rehearsal dinner with a last kiss before I would see him at the end of the aisle, and I had felt better about the whole thing. I didn't need to think about heart jumpies and dizziness; I only needed to think about my hands in his as we said our vows to each other. Now, the day of, I had reached a point of absolute Zen. I had control of the situation, my mind and my emotions. What a beautiful day.

"So when are you and Britt and Katrina going to have your hair done?" my father asked at ten o'clock that morning.

"Dad, Katrina is only nine. We're not paying for her to have her hair done. She can do it here. You knew that. You were supposed to arrange all of that. Britt and I, since she is my maid of honor, are just going." I started to feel the frustration build. After over a year of planning, some of these little details had slipped through the cracks. I guess I hadn't realized I would need to choreograph these kinds of things, too.

"Oh, she'll be so disappointed. I told her she was going with you."

"Dad, why would you do that?" I sounded exasperated. My Zen mellowness slipped a couple of notches.

"Well, she's your sister, for cryin' out loud!" He said, the anger and yelling escalating. "You can't just have your way and leave her out."

"SHE'S ONLY NINE! Do you have fifty dollars for someone to do her hair?" I knew that was a low blow because he didn't have any money for this sort of expense.

"DON'T BE SO SELFISH!" he countered.

"IT'S MY WEDDING DAY." I took a deep breath. "A little bit of help in some of the details about you guys could have been handled by you. I cannot do everything. Until this week, I wasn't even in the same STATE as any of this. I've been planning from afar, we've talked about plans every day, you KNEW that I had an appointment with Britt, so why would you try to throw this on me right as I'm getting ready to go, when there's not a chance that we can, or should, make it happen."

"Fine, Kat, do what YOU want to. I'll make sure Katrina gets her hair done. I wouldn't want to burden you." Oh my Lord. I can't believe we were arguing about something so crazy. I thought wedding days were supposed to be about bliss and family unity; not screaming and blaming. It's just the nerves, Kat. He's got them, too. It's all just a little overwhelming. I left and picked up Britt and we proceeded to have our hair done, putting the stress behind me. I looked forward to my wedding hair moment; so chic, so glam, so perfect.

"Since you have so much gray, I can't part your hair on the side like you want me to," the hair dresser said, causing a scratching halt of the record of little girl happiness turning in my head.

"What do you mean? I just colored it like a week ago." He snickered, which I found extraordinarily irritating and decided to instantly lower his tip.

"Sweetie, you're hair must grow really fast then, because you have a line of gray that's a half inch deep." He held a hand mirror up to my scalp and my eyes widened. Shit! How can a twenty-four year old have a solid gray, nay, shiny silver stripe dashing across her head? That's not right. And really not fair.

"What am I going to do? We don't have time to color it now."

"I could find a sharpie and color it in," he said, giggling sadistically to himself. That's it, no tip for him. "I'm just kidding, honey. I'll just have to sweep it straight back instead of pulling at the part. It'll still look fine." Great. Fine. That's the dream of every bride, right? How did you look at your wedding? Oh, you know, fine. Average. So-so. Thanks for asking. I sighed.

"Well, just do the best you can. My veil will make it all better. Hopefully nobody will notice that I turned sixty overnight." Okay, so things weren't going quite as smoothly as planned. I had heard horror stories about weddings and if this ended my problems, then I would be getting off easily. We paid; I even included a tip for salvaging the situation; had our make-up done, then headed back to my dad's to meet up with the other girls where we would rendezvous with the limo, send the maids over first, then have a final father/single daughter bonding moment as we headed to the church for the girls to get dressed there. Those were the plans. Instead, another scenario played out. But wouldn't you have guessed?

My sister came bounding out of the apartment when Britt and I returned and I hardly even recognized her. Her normally straight hair had been curled, teased, blown and sprayed into a pyramid of submission. Bangs and poufs and puffs of hair followed each turn of her head as if shackled in place. Each hair had clearly lost all sense of free will. Her eyes dazzled me like Liza Minnelli, her cheeks rouged like a Vegas showgirl and her lips as red as if stung by a menacing insect.

"Wow," I said, as she looked at me excitedly. "Wow." I heard Britt chuckle behind me.

"Don't I look pretty, Sissy?" I nodded with my eyes enlarged, not quite sure how to answer.

"Wow," I said again. The other girls arrived in one car at that moment, their dresses flung over their shoulders in rustling plastic garment bags. The limo drove by, then noticing all the women with nice hair, backed up. Yep, this is the place, big guy! All of this coincided with my father busting out of the front screen door in his underwear and socks, rage ablaze. He looked like a troll, an angry, unembarrassed Emperor's New Clothes fan. His graying tighty-whities hung loosely on his non-existent hips, saggy from overuse and over-washing.

"Where have you BEEN, Kat?"

"What are you talking about? Getting my hair and makeup done. Where do you think? Dad, go put some clothes on. You're supposed to be in your tux. The limo's here." I didn't even want to make eye contact with my maids. My father had shown this side of himself to many people, but right now and in front of these people, well, just seemed all wrong.

"I've been scurrying around trying to find someone to do your sister's hair and makeup, which your Aunt graciously offered to do, since you wouldn't take her. And your grandmother is here and she needed help getting ready."

"Now, David, I'm fine. I don't need your help," I heard my grandmother say from inside the house.

"How could you be so SELFISH, Kat, and leave me to figure all of this stuff out?" He screamed. A couple of neighbors stepped out onto their front porches, unused to a spectacle at this time of day, involving a bunch of people in a variety of stages of dress. We sure looked like a classy bunch.

"DAD, ALL I ASKED YOU TO DO WAS GET DRESSED! AND GET MY

SISTER DRESSED. THAT'S IT. FOR THE WHOLE DAY. AND WALK ME DOWN THE AISLE," I yelled.

"Well, I DON'T EVEN WANT TO DO THAT NOW!" he yelled back. I started to cry, messing up a perfectly beautiful makeup job from a makeup counter at the mall. The maids encircled me protectively, ushering me in the opposite direction of my father, providing a bridal shield against evil. They could have been superheroes. Britt, the maid of honor extraordinaire, took her duties a step further than requested and marched right up to my father with determination and Bitch in her eyes.

"Dave," she said, and I almost fainted because I'd never heard her call my father, who she had known since she was seven, by his first name. She pointed her finger right in his face. "Get your ASS back in that house and put your tuxedo on. This is your daughter's one and only wedding day. I will NOT stand here and let you ruin it. You have five minutes. Then you will get in that limo and you will not make her cry anymore. Get dressed NOW." He looked at her with fury, then burst out laughing, holding his hands up in surrender.

"Fine, I'm going. You guys are hilarious, like a bunch of little bees protecting the queen. Man, did she pay you for that?" But he went. And he got dressed. Meanwhile the maids left in the limo to the church, but not before making sure that I would be okay first. What wonderful maids. I realized though, that once they'd left in the limo that they'd forgotten my grandmother. She would now have to ride in it with us for our father-daughter moment when the limo returned to pick us up. I actually felt pretty good about this as I still smarted from having to cry on my wedding day from a stupid fight with my father. Grandma would get to play buffer.

The limo pulled back around and passed the house again. Geez, what was up with this guy and his sense of direction? He reversed when he realized that the man in the tux, old woman and girl with the veil needed a ride somewhere. My father opened the door, finally zipped up, fully clothed and gentlemanly. My grandmother took a step in and fell flat on her face. The poor woman was eighty and not very fit, so it took all of the effort of us and the driver to lift her back up enough to kind of slide her in head first and try to position her into a seat. Luckily she didn't hurt herself, but with the temperature hovering around ninety-five, we all broke a sweat. This was not a great look for a fresh bride, and my dad had to remove his jacket after just putting it on. He hated those things anyway, and I think secretly harbored resentment that I made him wear a tux with a dreaded tie to the wedding at all. Yet, somehow we all shifted into our seats and tried to enjoy the short trip to the church. I had expected a heartfelt little talk about moving from 'little girl' to 'woman', perhaps topped off with a small champagne toast; not a surly, glaring stare-off, interrupted by slight moans of pain from my bruised grandmother.

We arrived at the church and quickly separated to the boys and girls dressing rooms without so much as a word. I relaxed as my maids gathered all around me to offer touch ups and help me into my dress. I stood before the full length mirror and couldn't help but smile. Nothing else from the day mattered anymore. We existed only in the present. I wanted to be here, marrying the love of my life, in front of all of my friends and family. I felt better than I had in a long time. Maybe just this once I could try not to think about all of the possible health problems I might have, and just enjoy the moment. Of course, I was breaking the rule by even thinking that thought there, but at least the idea was in the right place.

The church coordinator lined us up, my navy blue maids ahead of me as we walked single-file to the foyer of the sanctuary. My father greeted me there to take my arm and lead me down the aisle. I caught his eye and all animosity disappeared; had never existed.

"And now we're calm," he said into my ear. "It's time to go down the aisle." He squeezed my arm gently before allowing me to link it through his own.

The organ played Pachabel's Canon and the maids stepped-stopped all the way to the front one at a time. My sister, designated as Junior Bride's Maid headed down right before Britt, a glowing beacon with cherry cheeks. As I walked down I looked from left to right slowly and noticed all the faces watching me with emotion; their happiness for me obviously tinged with sadness at the absence of my mother. We had noted an honor to her at the bottom of the program and the whole room felt her presence spiritually, heavily.

As we said our vows, I could hear the sniffling from all directions. There's not a dry eye in the house. The men are even crying. My heart skipped a few beats as we finished the standard vows and entered into the part of the program where we spoke to each other with our own words. Keep it together, Kat. Now's not the time to worry about your heart attacks, or hypoglycemia, or fainting spells. Now's the time to REMEMBER YOUR WORDS. I started to speak and a loud clap of thunder rang out, echoing throughout the church, masking over my words. When Jason spoke the thunder cracked and reverberated, bouncing off the pews and the balcony. God? Is that you? Are you trying to tell us something? Or is this just August in Orlando? We heard the beating rain, a sudden storm upon us, pounding the roof, overtaking not just our words, but the music accompaniment as well. I laughed in spite of myself and we could hear snickers from the audience, a relief from all the previous tear jerking. The minister pronounced us husband and wife; at least pronouncing our name correctly for the first time; we had so many issues during the rehearsal. As we stepped out onto the stairs at the entrance, the clouds parted and the sun beamed again. I've heard that rain on your wedding day can actually be considered good luck. But blasts of thunder and torrential rain during the all important vows followed by a total clearing of weather directly afterward, where it seemed like a direct path to heaven had opened up, well, it just seemed strange. Plus, the storm left us with an exorbitant amount of humidity.

The limo took the maids to the reception and would return to pick us up, giving us time alone for a few minutes as a couple and to have a few more pictures taken. When half an hour went by and he did not return, we got worried. When the church locked up the door and handed us our duffle bags, our concern grew. When the two of us stood alone in the parking lot and everyone had left completely, we wondered what the hell had happened. I mean, really, the bride and groom are missing. Didn't anyone remotely notice this? A custodian saw us standing there and offered a ride in her Geo Storm. Jason climbed into the back seat of the two door car. I hiked up my large white dress, sat down with a thump and smashed the fabric all around me to make it fit, like a lemon meringue pie squashed into a tiny Tupperware box. Just as our Storm came to life, the limo arrived, honking its horn.

"I'm sorry, I got lost." Are you effing kidding me? I mean after you've been lost twice at the same house and had already been to the church, what gives? Was this guy the worst with directions in the history of all mankind? It was approximately one turn and a straight road to get to the reception. Perhaps he had taken too much prescription medication. Perhaps he was just an idiot. Perhaps he should find a different career than driving limos. Either way, I could feel my pulse quicken. I would not let this fine gentleman ruin our big day. Cleansing breath. Deep cleansing breath. Let it go.

Once at the reception, I did let it go. I ate a finger full of icing, and not much else. I drank champagne, danced until my feet blistered, threw out my painful shoes in the trash, then danced some more. I spun around in my dress; beautifully handmade for me by the mother of one of my maids, adorned with pearls taken from an old necklace of my mother's. I hugged and held hands, greeted and loved. My baby sister gave a speech and unknowingly wished us good sex that evening.

"I hope they have a good time tonight and make babies."

All in all, I'd say the wedding day went quite well. I later found out, of course, that the air had not been turned on at the church in time and it felt like an oven right about until the time when I took a step down the aisle, so I didn't notice. The family who had my dress pressed for me brought it to the church that morning and the whole place had been locked up with no-one in sight. They had to track down strangers and finagle a way in through a mistakenly unlocked back door just to make sure my dress was there waiting for me when I arrived. Hey, every wedding needs a little dose of breaking and entering. We had run out of wine and someone had kindly gone out to get more. The church coordinator had forgotten to put the flowers and ribbon on the pews, so at the last minute, some guests had joined forces and decorated for us. But all of these things took place outside my line of vision. And the after-tales made me truly understand how blessed and loved I am and we are, as a couple. More than any other day, I learned that day to be grateful.

\*\*\*

We honeymooned in Europe, a two and a half week adventure comprised of Paris, then a train to Madrid for a couple of days, a train to Malaga on the Costa Del Sol for a week at the beach, a train to Barcelona for a couple more days, then a train back up to Paris to finish the journey. We would definitely learn the European rail system on this trip. What a spectacular adventure. In Paris, we dined on the Champs Elysee, kissed at the top of the Eiffel Tower, discovered the sweet mystery of pain au chocolat, and traversed the Louvre until we could take it no more and needed a café au lait. Bien.

When we took our first train to Madrid, we found ourselves in the second class car with no air, and it was boiling outside in August through the Spanish countryside. Although the signs said "No Fumar," people were fumaring all over the place, their lit cigarettes dangling out of their mouths as they spoke, not impeding their speech in the slightest. Meanwhile I gasped for air and considered how fast lung cancer could possibly develop. A sweaty soccer hooligan- I say this because he was loud and wearing a jersey from some Spanish team- walked past us, reached out, grabbed my lemon Fanta, took a swig with his swarthy, moist lips, then replaced it on my tray table. He said something in Spanish, and I looked to my husband for translation; he just shrugged, no help at all. I stared at my beverage, now a foreign, toxic specimen, grossed out by its general appearance, once so inviting and now so repellant. I silently prayed for the concessions cart to come through so I could at least get a little water. The blazing heat aimed to dehydrate me at its earliest convenience. I wanted to just let the hooligan know he could have the whole thing, as if he had sprayed like a cat. This can belonged to him; his territory, I would interfere no more. But he had moved on to sample other peoples' wares.

Once in Madrid, the first order of business was to secure a first class ticket for all remaining train rides. We found luck for the next short trip to Malaga, but the overnight from Malaga to Barcelona was booked so we would have to suffer through second class again. Okay, we guess we could make it, we told ourselves. We would just make sure we secured first class on the overnight back up to Paris. Thinking we had taken care of business, we set out to enjoy Madrid. The Prado, Spanish palaces, extraordinary paella and delicious sangria. Bueno. Outside of the transvestite prostitutes that graced the little cobblestone road of our hotel, or the loud Goth bar just outside of our hotel room, or that fact that my hair dryer created a short that threw the electricity out on our whole floor and we had to live in the dark for over a day, we LOVED Madrid. And when we had to leave, we loved the first class train ride to Malaga. We basked in the air conditioned car filled with trendily clad adults. We amored the food car with pretty little flowers on the tables, windows on the side and roof. Everybody on this train car adhered to the No Fumar signs. We had more than forgotten about our previous train encounter.

In Malaga we enjoyed watching the pasty British people in their Speedos and fanny packs on holiday, baking themselves into oblivion, resembling rotating pigs on a stick at a Luau. At one point we saw a gentleman with a pale potbelly, angry red nose and shoulders and a black fanny pack. It took us a long time to realize that he had a black Speedo underneath because the overhang of his stomach shadowed the lower area, hiding it from the world, only revealing the more obvious outer shell of the fanny pack. I know it's not polite to stare at the nether regions of someone's body, but his outfit, or lack thereof, was such a conversation piece. We wanted to lift the belly up ourselves to see if the Speedo was indeed truly under there. In addition to people watching, we went to a bullfight; cool culturally, but god awful gruesome and disgusting. I had not realized beforehand that I would repeatedly witness the stabbing and bleeding of the bull; and have to cheer for it. So gross. The next night, to block the startling images from my mind, I booked us for dinner at a Flamenco show, with a touch of Spanish ballet. That's more like it. The show offered a little more peace in my head. We also took the boat to Morocco from Gibraltar and viewed snake charming, fabulous architecture, and a large assortment of rugs we were aggressively pressured to purchase. We enjoyed this week of reprieve from the more active touring in the bigger cities but alas, we needed to board our next train.

Now, when we realized we would need to travel second class again, we figured we would suffer through the same sort of problems faced on the previous hooligan infested train; just overnight. Instead, Jason and I boarded the train, regarded our tickets, and only then noticed that we had tickets for two different second class cabins. That's honeymoon romance right there. He took me to mine first and when I walked in- rather, scooted and inched sideways through the extremely narrow door opening- into the closet they called a cabin; my eyes darted from the floor to the ceiling. The bunk beds were three deep on each side, and one woman also had a baby. Seven of us in a room no bigger than seven feet by five feet. And no air conditioning. And windows stuck in place as if super glued. I needed a paper bag, stat. I started to hyperventilate. The family, none of whom spoke English, of course, smiled at me and spoke, but I just weakly nodded and slipped right back out.

"I can't do that. I can't sleep in there. I'll just have to sit out here in the hall."

"Look, I know it's not ideal," Jason said, clearly frustrated at our dumbness for not realizing we needed to make reservations and that the Europass ticket did not suffice on its own for a good seat or room. "But let's just go to the dining car. We'll get a bite to eat, play some cards, and then you won't have to go back in there until it's time for sleeping. No worries. It's just one night." True. I guess I could handle that. It seemed rational at the time. I grudgingly followed him rather than my choice which involved leaping off the train and high tailing it to the nearest airport.

We lucked into our own table at the dining car and I order Salmon; a personal favorite at restaurants. People were fumaring everywhere, but I tried to breathe normally; though with each breath I imagined my lungs darkening and the carcinogens roaming. I also tried to think cooling thoughts to counteract the tremendous heat trapped on the train. We ate, but I could only take a few bites. When I get nervous, my stomach coils up like a rattle snake and can stay that way for hours or even days.

"Does this Salmon taste okay to you? It seems a little off to me." I said, pushing the fish towards Jason and nibbling on the rice on the side of the plate. Jason stuck his fork in, took a bite and declared it, "Fine." Of course, Jason has a stomach of steel. I have never seen him get sick from food. Me? I entertained nausea from food (too rich, too raw, too spicy, etc.) on a monthly basis at least, like a favored house guest. He ate the rest when he saw that I'd given up after about three small tastes. Oh well, I would just eat well in Barcelona. We played cards as promised and a little travel size Mancala. I whipped Jason's butt, but he would likely claim the opposite. Don't listen to him.

Finally a respectable time came to call it a night and try to sleep in my little tomb of too many people. Please let there be enough oxygen for all of us. I started to feel a little sick to my stomach, but again, I was tired, anxious and really sick of the Fumar! I kissed Jason goodnight and we parted ways; sad. I slipped into my cabin, slithered into my slot and tried to lay my head on my backpack as a pillow. Bang, I hit the bed above me. Apparently, my large head and backpack would not fit together in this suffocating space. Fabulous. I pushed the pack against the wall, looping my arm through one of the straps; in case anyone tried to steal the backpack, of course (hello, paranoia), and rested my head on the flat mattress, which resembled a real mattress in no way at all. I had no pillow. I closed my eyes and felt the rumbling of the train. The motion and noise ventured closer until I felt like I was part of the train itself. I opened my eyes and realized that part of the rumbling and noise came from my very own stomach. An agonizing pain shot through my midsection and climbed forcefully and volcanically up my body, into my esophagus. I leapt up, pounding my head into the darn bed above me again. A cold, very wet sweat broke out all over me and I started to shake. I grabbed my pack and dragged it quickly behind me. I didn't have the strength to lift it, as it felt much heavier than it had before bed. Or maybe I had weakened.

I barely made it into the bathroom before I threw up. Then in a wicked twist of fate, the sickness attacked the other end simultaneously. Oh the humanity. I reached for toilet paper to at least wipe my mouth, only to discover an empty dispenser. Stunned, violently sick, and crying my eyes out, I found myself on the ground of a public bathroom on a Spanish train for the next seven hours, repeatedly sick and without method of cleaning myself up. To make matters worse, I lived through this feeling on a train, which continued to move; vibrating, bouncing, and lurching from side to side. At this point, I forgot all about my honeymoon and just wanted to die. I couldn't move, didn't have the strength to get up at all. I had no water and all concessions had long ago closed. I wish I could have MacGyvered something out of the contents of my backpack, but I was depleted physically and emotionally; drained, dehydrated and spent. Periodically, someone would knock on the door, needing to use this one bathroom that existed for about four cars worth of people.

"Sorry, someone's in here," I would cry desperately. Please help me. Or just kill me. I am dying anyway. This is what it feels like to die. I didn't even have it in me to gather myself to find Jason; just seven hours of vomiting and sickness. Oh my goodness, do I even have to tell you how bad I felt? I would not wish this experience on my worst enemy. I had found a true form of torture and violation. By the time my train pulled into Barcelona, I believed that I had debased myself more than I would ever have thought possible. I finally opened the door, and quickly snuck down the hall so that the next person to use the facility would not see that I had caused the wreckage. I hastily found Jason and pulled him rapidly off the train and to the nearest spot with the fewest people to describe my night and see if he had any provisions that might aid my time of need. He did not. But he did buy me some crackers and a lemon Fanta. In case you haven't noticed, Fanta is my European beverage of choice; outside of wine, of course. I went to the nearest bathroom and tried to wash up as best I could, throwing away my underwear; not salvageable; nothing further to add to that. If I wanted to turn this lemon of a situation into lemonade, I would say that I have since always remembered to bring a change of clothes in my backpack, deodorant, toothbrush and little refresher wipes. Live and learn, people. Just a little tip for you. No extra charge.

My back ached and felt broken from the long period of strenuous retching, so we grabbed a cab to our hotel in Barcelona only to find that, for the first time ever in Europe, our hotel room would not be ready for another couple of hours. Our photo album from this trip features only a few pictures of me in this most glorious city. I look sad and humiliated, standing in front of a cathedral, in soiled clothes, frowning. I don't even make eye contact with the camera, afraid the lens will see what has become of me; what I have been reduced to. The rest of the Barcelona pictures have no people in them, as they all contain lovely architecture and historical sites that Jason saw when he ventured out alone and I stayed in bed recovering with back spasms for the next two days. A few self-portraits mingle with the buildings, as Jason photographed himself eating tapas by himself. I would not have a single meal for the whole two days in Barcelona. One day, I owe that city another visit. The photos are extraordinary.

I eventually started to feel better and the horrendous back pain faded. I had started contemplating the possibility of permanent and possibly lethal long-term damage. I had successfully rehydrated myself and could walk from one room to the other without shaking too much; just in time to board the next train. With much trepidation, we embarked on the fast overnight train to Paris and discovered that we had our own luxury cabin. We're not sure how much extra we actually paid for it and don't care; it was worth every penny, or franc, at the time. This cabin had regular bunk beds, just two, our own private bath, equipped with shower, sink, lots of toilet paper and even bathrobes and slippers. I had known, or been pretty sure, I was going to die in the hell of the previous ride, and now I felt like I had been lifted to a light fluffy cloud somewhere in the suburbs of heaven. In the dining car, fully air conditioned and non-smoking, I carefully chose a nice pasta dish. No more salmon, an unfortunate rule that still applies to this day. I can't eat it, or even smell it for that matter; as if it had given me a bad tequila hangover. I have my salmon hangover.

Back in Paris, I felt renewed, refreshed and ready to eat Nutella crepes in the Jardin Toulleries. I found my back giving me permission to enjoy the Moulin Rouge; can-can, topless women and miniature ponies. Tres Magnifique! We finished off the honeymoon with flourish and much more dignity on my end. I stopped worrying about dehydration and spontaneous lung cancer. I stopped taking my pulse to make sure it beat at a normal pace. As we flew home, a ray of sunlight peaked in through my half-closed window shade and caught my diamond ring, sending a bright glare in my eyes. I angled my hand back and forth, stretching my arm for a better look (typical girl stuff), and I looked over at Jason, his eyes closed, head resting back. I felt at peace. I knew that I didn't usually have much inner peace with all the crap playing in my head all the time. But for this moment, this one fleeting moment, nothing scared me. I did not worry about death.

Hypochondriac Lesson #17:
Don't worry about the things you can't change.

*17- Baby's Growing Up*

"I don't have time to explain everything to you, so just get acclimated and see what you can learn on your own." Right before the door slammed, I heard him yell, "And ask questions. Just not any stupid ones." Well I guess I better rip up that list of dumb questions I was making. I now introduce you to my Boss of my first real career job. Rather than practice law, I ventured into the equally hated and loved field of professional fundraising, or as we like to refer to it in the inner circles, Development. I stared at the bare white walls of my new office and tried to figure out what exactly my job would entail as a fundraiser for the University without further irritating Boss. I knew I would need to ask people for money, but my knowledge ended there. Stupefied after Boss's sudden exit, I ran my hand across my desk and wondered how to progress. I liked having my own desk, felt like such a grown-up, but maybe I should have seen the signs that working for Boss would be a little different, to put it nicely.

When I had applied for the job, I had not expected to hear back so soon after sending in my resume, especially because I had no "development" experience. I had hoped my degrees would prepare me, but I had my doubts about this job. I almost jumped with excitement when Boss asked me to come in for an interview the morning after I had forwarded the resume to him. I had taken my one non-maxed credit card, a by-product of life as a student with no actual money, and went to an outlet mall outside the city to purchase a new suit for the interview.

I had startled awake in the morning before my alarm went off with nervous flitting in my abdomen. Heart jumpies commenced, like preschoolers doing jumping jacks, arms and legs everywhere with no discernable rhythm. I brushed my hair back into a smart and sophisticated bun and donned my new simple black suit, with lavender silk shirt peeking out from underneath. I strung a single strand

of small pearls around my neck, the necklace I had worn on my wedding day, for

good luck, to match the pearl studs in my ears. I spread a subtle taupe eye shadow

across my lids and applied mascara with slightly shaking hands. I'd been shaking a

lot lately. Parkinson's? Some other neurological disease? I wanted to do well, so I

needed to get past this.

I reveled at the chance to live in Nashville again. I had fallen in love during my

college days with the Southern charm and lively vibe that infused the city, with the

funky cafes, surprisingly decent bookstores, and especially the artsy coffee shops.

When eating at my favorite local pancake joint and gorging myself on cinnamon

spice pancakes, I loved that the waitress, an older lady with a heavy accent who

slowly drawled her words, didn't even have to write my order down. The sweet

tea of pretty much every restaurant practically gave me an orgasm. I had found

that Music City was not just all about country music- hopefully I do not offend,

but I can't stand most country music; the twang, the whine; not my bag- but

about all music. The city also graciously made room for numerous other cultural

pastimes, some that would rival any of the supposedly more cosmopolitan cities.

It had great hospitals; a consideration when deciding to move back. I adored the

infamous "Batman" building, its dual radio towers on either side of the structure

resembling the Dark Knight's costume ears (luckily no nipples). I tangibly felt the

hopefulness of the city. Nashville seemed to draw wanderers and artists, as if by

gravity, to start a new life, maybe get discovered and showcase their talents. While

I couldn't personally carry a tune; in fact, people requested specifically for me

to stop singing if they heard me; I related to these souls, even if I didn't sport the

seemingly obligatory cowboy hat, spangly outfit, or obscenely large belt buckle. I

couldn't wait to try to prove myself. This interview would be my own audition and

I wanted to get the chords and melody just right, so that I could embrace this new beginning of my life.

The secretary outside Boss's office had offered a warm, sincere smile as I entered the front door. In her mid-fifties, the woman came off as relaxed and breezy with her graying blond hair clipped up in a loose French twist and a casual navy blazer and knee-length skirt adorning her plump physique. I felt like I could quickly engage this woman in a heart-to-heart conversation and easily receive sympathy or delight in return depending on the circumstances. The woman rose and quickly moved around her desk, extending her hand to greet me.

"You must be Kat," she had said. "We're so excited to meet you. You come to us with glowing recommendations from the higher-ups," she said, pointing a finger from her other hand gently up in the air. She looked me over. "You seem a little nervous, honey. Relax; the Boss is going to love you. I can already tell. I've seen the people who've come and gone through here and I have a pretty good sense of what he's looking for when it comes to sending people out to our donors. And I'd say you certainly fit the bill." She looked approvingly at my outfit and hair. Thank the Almighty for my credit card and Casual Corner outlet. "So why don't you just take a seat here and keep me company. He'll be out in a jiff." I had smiled, relaxing a little, suddenly aware of how tense my posture had been and trying to slow my heart. I took the proffered seat across the desk from her and crossed my ankles, attempting all signs of ladylike behavior. I barely managed to sit back in the chair completely when Boss came bounding out of his office, flushed red in the face as if his office thermostat might be set ten degrees too high. Is he okay? He's either angry, hot, having a heart attack, or incredibly sunburned.

I guessed Boss's age as mid to late forties. He had thinning dark brown hair that seemed slightly disheveled. The hair was matched by a rumpled, wrinkled seersucker suit a couple of sizes too large for his body. I wagered that he'd recently lost weight, and not being very fashion-forward, failed to buy clothes to fit his new frame. I should've suggested the outlets I went to. His face appeared above the distracting clothes with green eyes and large ears that protruded slightly from his head. He was not particularly tall, yet he filled up the room with his presence. As with a stray dog, I could not decide with the first impression if he was entirely friendly. I had a mind to reach my hand out to let him sniff.

"Kat, yes?" He asked, gruffly. "Why don't you come on in with me here and let's get started. Hold my calls." Secretary nodded her assent at his command and I followed him into his office.

I had stepped into the room and immediately noticed the striking decor. Where the walls in the front office had been simple white and pretty typical of other middle management offices I had seen before, Boss's walls and furniture came straight out of a book of interior design. A plum-colored plush couch faced opposite to his desk, flanked by two beautiful Victorian chairs. Lush potted plants filled the corners and soothing, slightly exotic artwork covered the warm caramel-colored walls. Ornate lamps added texture and interest to the end tables on either side of the couch and a beautifully rich oriental rug covered most of the floor adding a colorful glow to the room. To me, it looked more like a private office or library in an upscale home rather than an office for a fundraiser at a university. I couldn't help but be impressed and noticed that this decor likely cost far more than all the furniture in our new apartment. Honestly, that's not saying a whole lot. But do fundraisers make this much money? If so, then SWEET! However, the décor seemed to directly contradict the man himself.

"So Kat," Boss had started, his color returning back to a normal shade and his speech falling into a friendly southern drawl, drawing my attention away from my surroundings and back to the task at hand, "tell me, why are you here?"

"Excuse me?" I suddenly felt a heat rise up my neck. Um, to get a job. Am I in the right place?

"Why, if you got your law degree, are you not headed off to a firm? Or even to practice?" He grinned at me, putting me on the spot and having a good time doing so.

"Well, I lost my mother quite unexpectedly a few years ago, and recently my father has had a number of health issues. My priorities have changed a bit." I paused to get my bearings. "I'm excited about going into fundraising because these events have caused me to evaluate what I really find important, and I want to do some good in the world. Life is short and I want to work hard and do something I'm passionate about and still get to see my family." It sounded a little rehearsed, but even though I had practiced this response, I genuinely meant every word. Since nobody could understand why I wouldn't practice, I had to face this question quite a bit.

"Hmm," he replied. "So money's no longer a driving factor to you, then?" Wow, brutal. Man gets right to the point.

"Well, I would sure like to say that it doesn't matter at all," I had responded, "but let's be honest. I wouldn't be doing anyone any good if I can't pay rent and support my family. I'm newly married and I have student loans. A lot of student loans. So money has to play a little bit of a role in my decision making."

"Good point. And I didn't say that pursuing money was necessarily a bad thing." Okay, then I AM pursuing money. Do you want to pay off my law school debt?

"I guess I've learned that people perform better if they're happy with what they're doing," I said, to close the deal.

"You seem to have had quite a few life lessons for someone so young."

"Oh, well," I said, shifting uneasily, "it's not all by choice, I can assure you. I'm trying to find the positive aspects of these incidences so I can move forward with success in my life."

"Fair enough," he said, seeming to back off a bit. He had been leaning forward on his elbows, Larry King style. He put his hand up in the air to indicate that I need not say anymore. "Why don't you tell me a little about your work and class experiences instead and we can see how those might work in your favor for this profession."

We talked for half an hour and I went through my resume and achievements, trying to win him over and convince him that I fit the bill for the position. He offered no real encouragement throughout the conversation and was generally hard to read. He downright frowned most of the time, and appeared annoyed the rest. He finally looked at me thoughtfully, tapping his index finger against his lips. Then he had sighed and put both hands on his desk as if he might get up suddenly. He had stared at me intensely with a hard-to-read seriousness. Is he disappointed? Bored?

"I like you, Kat," he had said, finally.

That was unexpected.

"I think you're straightforward and sincere. Donors like it when you're direct with them. But you also seem to be at ease with people and I like that. You see, when you meet these people, you have to woo them, befriend them, remind them about how wonderful this university is, and make them want to give you the money. It's all about relationships. They already know why you're visiting with them but they need to trust you." He paused, continuing to evaluate me for a reaction. "Sometimes you don't ask them for anything until you have met them

face-to-face a couple of times. If that's what it takes." He stopped and assessed
me, searching for any signs of fear, I'm sure. He drummed the fingers of one hand
rhythmically on his desk.

"But I think you might have it, you know, the ability to connect with people.

"Oh, thank you very much," I said. But Boss held up his hand so as not to be
interrupted, and looked at me sternly. Oops. Note to self, do not EVER interrupt
this man.

"I've been doing this for seventeen years and I have donors who call me all the
time with issues or just wanting to talk or meet for lunch. It's a wonderful system
and it breeds loyal support for the school."

"Really? You have donors who just want to see you, for you?" People really
choose to spend time with this man?

"Sometimes. Depends on the donor, of course. But it can be part of the deal.
What do you think? How're you feeling about this?" Confused, elated, like I may
throw up.

"Honestly, it sounds perfect and I can't wait to start."

He had laughed at my assumption, but nodded his head. "Then I think we have
a job to give you. We've been without a second-in-line for a couple of months now
and there are hundreds of potential donors starved for attention. It's time to start
tapping those resources. I want to get you out there right away."

I almost squealed like a small child with delight, but contained myself and
kept a relatively dignified, professional appearance more suitable to my age.
We can afford the apartment. We can afford food. Toilet paper. Heck, maybe a
newspaper subscription. Now we're getting crazy! This is a great day.

"I can start as soon as possible."

"We'll look forward to having you, then, Kat." He abruptly got up to shake my hand, and I stood to reciprocate. He ushered me out and shut the door behind me. Well that was abrupt, but who cares? I just got my first jo-ob!

\*\*\*

Now well into my first day on the job, I looked around and tried to muster that same excitement. Already the attitude in the office had changed, and I felt a bit like an interloper. Unsure what to do, I started by accessing the university network and database of donors. My security process had been complicated as the school had an obligation to ensure that nobody from the outside could easily log into the database and retrieve personal and financial information about alumni and donors. Befitting a prominent university, many alumni tended to have high incomes and could easily be found in society pages, Fortune 500 companies and newspaper features on a regular basis. Because of the accumulation of wealth and fame, the development staff kept files on the potential donors including pictures, article clippings and notes of conversations and visits made with them. Before I would ever sit down face-to-face with a donor, I would know a great deal about their family, business and hobbies. I felt like a stalker.

"Don't be stupid about this. You have to stroke their ego a little and really make them feel good about themselves. The better they feel, the more they give," Boss taught me. As the days progressed, he tended to pop in on random occasions and spout folksy wisdom at me like a taller version of Jiminy Cricket, but I made a point of storing each nugget as a mental note. He was certainly the type to give a pop quiz. He shouted at me and never restrained his annoyance if I came into his office for anything and didn't have a pad and pencil in case he decided he wanted to tell me something, even if I came in to ask HIM a question.

He gave me a list of over one hundred names that I should consider "my" donors to nurture and solicit for funds. Some of these donors were targeted for huge one-time gifts to fund buildings or scholarships. Others I would need to ask for smaller yearly contributions.

"I'll give you a little time with these. Then we will role play," he said ominously. I swallowed and nodded. What have I gotten myself into?

I studied the records of the donors on my list, attempting to absorb information and insight into the lives of these strangers that I would soon hopefully get to know personally. Previous development officers who had worked on them had keyed in pages of notes. I was startled to read in great detail about one woman's breast cancer treatment and another man's estranged relationship with his oldest son. I learned of job promotions of men in high-powered corporate positions and monetary values of their divorce settlements. I read about trust funds, money left to widows, business failures, untimely deaths and multiple marriages. I felt like I was spying on the secret lives of the rich and famous, or reading the National Enquirer; except these people had freely given over this information to a listening ear. I couldn't help but wonder if they had any idea that this many details about their lives sat recorded in a computer database. I couldn't imagine having such information on my own life written down and recorded without knowing about it.

"I know it seems weird, Kat," Boss said, pontificating on the subject as usual without letting me respond. I had learned quickly that he really enjoyed hearing himself talk. "But if you don't know this kind of stuff in advance, then you run the risk of insulting them if you don't ask the right questions. It's better to know that they've gone through an ugly divorce, than to ignorantly ask about their spouse. See? Can you imagine how much of a moron you would be if you did that? And if you know things that interest them, it's generally easier to talk to them. It's a winning situation all around." He stared at me to make sure I comprehended.

He often looked at me as if he thought I was a vacant vessel to be filled with his accumulated wisdom. Yes, I think I understand, Boss, but sometimes my small mind doesn't let me understand all these big words. There were so many things I would've loved to say openly.

"They would find it a waste of time for some naive little fundraiser to walk into their office and start asking a bunch of questions that she should already know the answer to and expect them to fork over large amounts of cash. It's like a dance and each person is supposed to know their part for it to work. It hurts if you step on their toes. Don't step on their toes, Kat. Learn to dance properly." He looked at me, irritated, as if searching to see the light of comprehension suddenly come on. "They know why you're there, Kat. Nobody has ever been surprised when a fundraiser comes to see them and then asks them for money. You seem afraid. Are you afraid?"

He instructed me as if I should have known everything all along. He phrased it as if the machinations of fundraising were common sense to everyone. Don't get me wrong, despite his patronizing manner, I felt like I learned something new every day. But I couldn't help but wonder if he talked like this to his donors. Surely not. He targeted the really big dollars and while a candid touch was good, I was sure, his behavior sometimes bordered on obnoxious. I had heard him shout vulgarities to other university employees then slam the phone down, cursing under his breath, but not really attempting to hide his hostility. Then he would quickly morph into the laid back southern gentleman like he had been for a bit during my interview. I came to see that there were two very different sides of the man, each requiring healthy respect. If I wanted to gain his knowledge, I needed to be wary of the pendulum swing of his moods, and try not to get on his bad side; at least, more on his bad side. Everyone was already on his bad side. You couldn't avoid the bad side.

"If they don't like you, Kat, they won't help you out. I can guarantee that. That's what the relationship aspect is all about. Make them want you. Use yourself to bring in the dollars." Now that just made it sound like I'm a prostitute.

Feeling a bit awkward with my stark white walls and generic office furniture compared to the warm and plush environment of Boss's office, I took a little time to hang my framed degrees and some inexpensive watercolor prints I picked up at a local craft store. I placed a vase of flowers on my desk and hoped that I'd created at least a little bit more pleasant of an environment. Boss peered in one day and gave an approving nod as he gave the space a quick once-over.

"This is a good start, Kat. I mean, clearly not finished." Oh. I looked around the office. "We need to always put on a good face and offer an inviting place for people if they come by the office. By the way, I've been meaning to tell you that I like your wardrobe. Subtle jewelry, close-toed shoes. Very polished, conservative. Some of these girls that have come through here tend to think this is a fashion show. And while it's good to be stylish, I guess, just remember that we're dealing with some rich folks in their sixties and seventies who have no interest in purple toenails or whatever the hell's in style these days. Just watch the use of sandals, even if it's warm." He quickly disappeared without waiting for a response. Wow. Okay.

I always dressed simply and as sophisticated as my budget allowed; even if I tended to wear the same few items with much frequency. It was strange to have someone blow in, scrutinize my clothes unexpectedly and quickly retreat without warning. I was starting to notice a pattern with Boss and his impromptu visits to my office that were brief, sudden and loud. He was a gunshot. Once the echo of his voice died down as he exited the room, I was often left stunned and confused about what just happened.

After a few weeks on the job, taken up mostly by researching, Boss started pressing me to set up appointments to visit some donors. The idea made me a little anxious. Calling people I had never met before to try to get into their offices and homes seemed so intrusive to me. I attributed it to my status as a novice in the field, but I felt clueless and in serious need of a little more guidance. All the research in the world wouldn't help me in the actual moment if I was antsy, sick to my stomach, worried about heart failure, and didn't know what to do. I hesitantly broached the subject with Boss.

"Would it do some good for me to accompany you on a visit or two just to see how you go about it?" I asked one morning, feeling like a toddler for even broaching the question. "Strategies, that kind of thing. It would be great to see an example of how you move a conversation along to get it to where you want it to be," I said. I couldn't help but notice his frown emerge.

"You could come with me, Kat, sure, but really the best way to learn how to do it is just to do it, if you know what I mean," he said, with slight disapproval, as if I was silly for not inherently understanding that. "Here's the thing, Kat," he pressed on, "each of these appointments is completely different. It's better just to go with your gut and determine when the time is right to pounce, okay? But I'll give you one piece of advice. When you do get around to asking for the dough, make the ask, then shut up." He paused, as if demonstrating the technique. "If you keep talking, they have an easier time avoiding what you just asked them for and will steer the subject away from the matter at hand. And nobody wants to hear you talk."

"But…"

"Kat, please don't interrupt me." Oh for crying out loud. He looked around;

hoping something in the room would trigger his brain to what he'd been saying. "Oh, yes, also, you need to ask them for the right amount. They might be insulted if you ask for too much. But you also don't want to shortchange yourself, and let them get away with giving less than what you know they might if you had been better at your job. So basically, pick up the phone and start earning your keep." He smiled at me, a cat-about-to-eat-a-fish smile, and I sensed that he was only half joking. No pressure.

"Listen, I get what you're saying. It's just…" I tried not to look at his face contorting in anger. "I think it would be good for me sit in on a visit anyway just to get an idea of actually how to tell someone that I want money from them. In many cases, a lot of money. I want to see an example," I said. Then, seeing his red coloring, rushed on, "even if all the visits will be different." I watched him breathing, deeper than normal breathing. Is he going to explode?

"Fine," he said eventually. "But just know that you'll probably end up feeling ridiculous sitting there silently while the donor and I have a pleasant conversation." Then I will just have to feel ridiculous.

Meanwhile, on the home front, my time had arrived for my annual womanly check up and I went to white-knuckle my way through the appointment. I had only been to a few of these in my life, but to be fair, detested each one equally. I broke out into a cold sweat on the day I made the appointment, and then anticipated its arrival with fear, trepidation and terrible digestive problems each day in between. When I entered the office, I had to excuse myself right away to go to the restroom for impending sickness. The nurses raised their eyebrows when reading my blood pressure- lab coat blood pressure victimized with its wicked pincers- and opened their mouths slightly when attempting to count my pulse. I only made it through this messy endeavor by remembering that the whole appointment only lasted a couple of minutes. And, as I noted before, I liked this hospital.

The doctor, and med school student in training, conducted my exam. When they started the circular motions with two fingers on my breasts to check for lumps, the doctor frowned. Now, let me clear something up here; as an aside. When a doctor frowns at me or whatever body part he happens to be touching at the time, I do not appreciate it. I don't want to see my doctor frown, look shocked, look perplexed, look upset. I want to see nothing. All normal, nothing to see here. Wham, bam, you have a clean bill of health, go. So when she frowned at me, then grunted a question mark, my heart decided to take flying lessons, and apparently liked them.

"What is it?" I asked, weakly, sickly.

"It's probably nothing. And over eighty percent of the time, they are benign. But I feel a mass that I would like to get checked out. I'm going to refer you to radiology for a sonogram just to make sure." Mass? Radiology? Well, if the mass doesn't kill me, I might just go ahead and die right now.

"Wh-what?" I might have just had a stroke. I immediately started to cry, blubbering out words that they may or may not have understood. "Buw, I jus got married!" I sobbed, barely comprehensible to myself, my voice squeaking so high, and interlaced with too many breaths. I verged on hyperventilation. "I can't have cancer." I wanted them to just tear off my breast right then. Who needs it? Jason loved me. He would have to love me without my cancer-infested breast.

"Calm down," said the doctor, putting her kind bedside manner to good use. The intern, on the other hand, looked horrified (he needed to work on that), and took a couple of steps backwards. "Like I said, it's likely nothing, but I just want to be on the safe side. I don't want you to worry about it." I wept while she talked, although nodding my head that I understood. Then I continued to weep as I left the building. I wept as I got in my car and I wept all the way home. I controlled myself as I called in sick to Boss for the rest of the day, then wept as I called Jason and told him that his twenty-four year old new bride now stood at death's door.

"People get lumps all the time," Jason said. "You can't worry about it until they tell you it's something to worry about. And they told you to specifically NOT worry about it." I wept. "When's your appointment for the sonogram?"

"Not for a month! How am I supposed to stay sane until then?"

"Just try to forget about it until then." What did he know? He didn't have a tumor.

I didn't forget about it. Every day I contemplated my fate. I started to look online at wig sites and read all about chemotherapy and radiation and surgery and recovery. I was sure I could feel it growing in my breast, an alien taking over my body and turning me into something unfamiliar. I looked up local support groups. I would need all the support I could find to go through what I knew lay ahead.

Meanwhile, Boss wanted me to start going on donor visits. I knew I had to carry on with life until my demise, but I couldn't seem to muster the energy to care. Perhaps the cancer had already started to sap my energy levels. Finally, I could hold out no longer. I made the calls. Maybe if I could focus on my work for a little bit, I could divert my attention away from tragedy. Besides, I couldn't lose my job, in case of survival.

The day of my first donor visits arrived quickly and coincided with my breast sonogram. I would have my donor visits then head to the radiologist in the afternoon. I stayed late the previous two days to prepare for the donors, making sure all files and notes were in order and trying to memorize as much about the two men I would see as possible. Boss cornered me that morning to give some last minute tips, although I found his delivery curt and grumpy, as usual.

"Look, Kat, try not to come across as a scared little girl," he said. I saw spittle. "Remember that this is a conversation you're having with them. So don't take notes or anything stupid like that. For Christ's sake, get out there and stand up to these people. Make them love you. Then the university will get to see the love, okay?" He really does think I'm stupid. And why does he have to be so mean? Can't he see that I'm dying here?

I stared at him for a second in disbelief, then gathered my things and thanked him as sincerely as possible for the advice, trying to stay composed from his caustic remarks, before brushing past him and heading confidently, as far as he could see, out the door.

I'm not sure how I did it, but I managed to convince one man to give the school forty thousand dollars and another to commit five thousand a year for five years. I had done it. I had managed professional success the first time out. Eureka! I had talked to the men, sharing stories about the school we all loved and they had been so kind, so gracious about my visit. I had been sucker-punched by the checks that they so easily wrote and handed over to me. For a brief moment, I felt on top of the world. Then I remembered my next stop.

I anxiously approached the door to Radiology at the University's hospital. I took a deep breath, and opened it, hoping my heart wouldn't stop before I could even enter. I could hardly breathe as I signed in and took my seat. My mouth had dried up and I had difficulty swallowing without saliva. My hands inadvertently played with each other, slick with sweat. That must be where the saliva disappeared to. I glanced furtively around the room, not wanting to stare, but just to see who had to go through this heartache with me. I came face-to-face with my future as my eyes landed on a woman with a colorful silk scarf wrapped around her bald head. I saw four or so women who appeared over the age of sixty, which made a little more sense to me, but then also saw another woman sitting with fear, absent-mindedly pushing a baby stroller back and forth, sadness full in her eyes. I tried to take more deep breaths. After a while, the door opened and a nurse came out.

"Kat Spitzer," she said, looking at the clipboard, then up to the waiting room crowd. I jumped up, my heart flip-flopping in my chest, and my hands shaking as I picked up my purse. She smiled. "This way through here." I followed her into a dark room where she made me change into the gown "open side to the front" and lie down and wait for the technician. I changed as fast as my quaking self would allow me and hopped up onto the bed, paper cover crunching menacingly underneath me as I tried to situate myself. Is this what mom felt like when she was about to die?

After what seemed like hours, but was probably closer to ten minutes, the technician came in and told me to put my arm up as she squeezed the warm jelly onto my breast and started prodding around with the sonogram instrument. I could tell when she found the lump because she started moving slowly around one particular spot, stopping periodically to type with one hand on the computer, while still holding the piece on my breast. She measured and froze frames so that all the necessary information would be available for the doctor to review. I tried to read her face but she gave nothing away.

"Is everything okay?" I asked. Please just tell me something before I vomit all over you.

"I'm sorry; I'm not supposed to say anything. I just take the pictures. The doctor will look it over and get back to you."

"When will that be?"

"Oh, she'll do it right after this. You'll know if there's a problem before you leave today."

"Does there look like there's a problem?" Maybe if I just kept trying? She just

looked at me and smiled, like no way, sister, your tricks won't work on me. Fine,

be that way. She finished up after only a couple of physically painless minutes

and gave me a couple of paper towels to clean up the lava flow of goo oozing

all over my breast. I waited for another eternity; maybe another ten or fifteen

minutes. I jumped again as the door opened and braced myself for the news, my

eyes squinting like I stood before a firing squad and not a pleasant looking doctor

wearing a sweater.

"Everything looks fine." Whoosh, I blew out all the pent up air in my lungs.

The angels started singing and I just knew that a blue sky and chirping birds waited

for me outside. "You have a simple cyst." Whoa, hold up. I have a cyst? Aren't cysts

bad? "This cyst is a perfectly round sack, not connected to anything. It moves

around and is filled with clear fluid. It is not anything to worry about and will

probably just go away on its own. If it starts to get painful, we can do a needle

aspiration, but my guess is that it will just go away." Oh, okay. "So you're okay."

I continued to stare at her. "You don't have anything to worry about." It finally

registered. I know she could see the palpable relief wash over my face. I wanted to

hug her, but restrained myself. Might as well keep some form of dignity.

I left the building, wanting to shout, "I'M ALIVE. I DON'T HAVE CANCER."

I fully expected all the flowers to be in bloom suddenly and maybe the munchkins

to come out of their hiding places like in the Wizard of Oz and sing me a song of

encouragement and celebration. I called Jason immediately and he said, "See, I told

you there was nothing to worry about." Fine. Know-it-all. Hooray. I'm queen of

the world, and, now that I could shift my focus, a Development Rock Star.

When I arrived back at the office, I expected to see Boss and share the good news- about the donors, he knew nothing about the cancer scare- but Secretary informed me that he'd already left for the weekend. I was so excited about my acquisitions that I had to share it with someone, so I filled her in on the donor visit details.

"Wow, great job, that's practically unheard of your first time out alone! Boss is going to be really happy about that."

"You think?" I asked.

"Listen, Honey, I probably shouldn't tell you this," she whispered, looking around as if expecting eavesdroppers. "Professionalism and all that. But in case you haven't figured it out, Boss is not exactly the easiest person to work for." She chuckled to herself, stating the obvious. "In fact, you're the fourth new person in this position in two years." My eyes widened in surprise and she nodded reassuringly. "I can tell you've been a little, um, startled by his way of handling things. But that's just how he is. Don't take it personally. I think that's where your predecessors went wrong. When he called them idiots, they got upset. He's like that with everyone he works with. He's even been known to shout at the higher-ups."

"I've heard him do that a couple of times actually," I said, relieved to hear her share the evidence.

"Haven't you noticed how red he gets?" She laughed again. "Looks like a tomato. He brings that my way sometimes, but I just put up my hand and let it roll off my back and I know you can too. I think he really does like you and I know he thinks you're doing a good job. Especially once he hears about today. So just hang in there and try not to let it stress you out or get you down. And you should know that he's nothing like that with his donors. The little old ladies absolutely adore him. Mmm hmm. He knows how to pour on the charm, and he's damn good at raking in the cash. I think that's why the bosses overlook his management style, to use the term loosely." She looked at me, appraisingly. "If you can stick it out, you might be surprised by how much you can learn from him. That is, if he'll let you." She chuckled again but looked at me earnestly. I had underestimated her awareness.

"Thank you. You have no idea how good it is to hear you say all that. I've been worried that I was just imagining it or that I was doing something really wrong. I mean sometimes his behavior is weird, right?" She nodded her head. "But geez, four people in two years is an awful lot. I don't feel so bad. I can understand why I sometimes get the impression from him that he doesn't expect me to last."

"Well, honey, all I got to say is, you prove him wrong." She winked at me then resumed her work, as if the conversation had never occurred. Just between the ladies.

Hypochondriac Lesson #18:
You are stronger and more awesome than your fear.

## *18- Moving Up During a Downer*

"Kat, wake up. Wake up! Come quick. A plane just flew into the World Trade Center. You won't believe this. Some idiot has flown his plane into the side of the building." Jason tried whispering so as not to startle me awake, but of course, that didn't work. The rapid shaking of me did the trick, hushed, hissing yell or not. I groaned, but managed to roll over and confront the tower of boxes looming on my side of the room, taunting me. *You think you can just keep walking around us, ignoring us, but we'll just keep getting in your way, until we block the door completely and you won't be able to get out unless you jump out your seventh floor window. Ha ha*, they said to me, leering at me with their brown three-dimensionality and layer of moving truck dust.

I stumbled out into the living room of the tiny new apartment in Arlington we had moved into; rather, unloaded into, as it would take eons to unpack anything and actually move into this space. We had taken jobs in Washington D.C. and stepped into our apartment on September 9, 2001. I yawned as I stumbled into the small space in front of the TV and sat on a box to see what Jason felt compelled to wake me up to witness.

"What kind of moron would not see the tallest structure in New York right in front of him?"

"What kind of plane is it?" I asked, casually. Interesting story, but I could have heard about it after I brushed my teeth and maybe had breakfast. We'd been up so late trying to just arrange the boxes so we could walk around. There actually seemed to be more boxes than space. It was tough to know exactly where to begin. I rotated my arm in a big circle to stretch out my sore shoulder.

"I don't know, it's hard to tell. Look at all that smoke. It can't have been too

small a plane. I wonder why the pilot was flying so low in that area to begin with."
Then, "What the fuck?!" We watched the footage of the second plane fly into the
second building of the World Trade Center and we stared at the screen, totally
speechless.

"Oh my god, that was no accident," I said, stating the unbearable obvious. The
smoke billowed on the screen and I felt the growing sick in the deep cavern of my
stomach. Fear. Devastation for the people experiencing firsthand what I watched
on TV, mere hours away by car or train. But mostly a general growing terror. It
crept through my body like a vine, wrapping its new growth around organs and
blood vessels, continuing its journey up into my throat where it twisted tightly
waiting to bloom out of my mouth. I quickly ran to the bathroom. I wanted to
watch to see what would happen, but at the same time, couldn't watch because the
images curdled my insides.

"What's wrong with you?" Jason asked. "This doesn't affect you." He was
trying the usual tactic to keep me settled, but I could hear the strain in his voice.

"We just moved to D.C. If something like that can happen in New York, don't
you think it could happen here? The President lives here. Besides, we could know
someone in those buildings." The reality suddenly hit me. "DO we know anybody
in those buildings?"

"Calm down. Nobody is going to attack Washington D.C. Do you know how
protected the air space is around here?" No. "This is a freaky, isolated incident and
we don't know the reason for it yet. No worries. Now let's think about if we do
know anyone in those buildings." Always the calm one. We started listing people
we knew in New York, who luckily didn't work anywhere near the buildings. But
as we racked our brains, we heard a massive sound of sirens and alarms as truck
after truck, rescue vehicle after rescue vehicle flew past our patch of high rise

buildings. I shot Jason a look of utter horror.

"Something's happened," I said. He didn't respond, just went silent and watched the TV for an answer. Within minutes the anchor reported that a fire blazed at the Pentagon, just down the street from us. Shortly thereafter, we learned that a third plane had crashed into the Pentagon. I ran back into the bathroom, only this time, Jason didn't question my actions. He felt the fear and pain as well. Over the next minutes and hours, we heard reports of a fire at the Capitol, and lock downs and fires at the Department of Justice and other government buildings. Questionable reports circulated about the state of the White House. We tried to make phone calls but the wires, even cell phone signals, had all crossed and twisted and nobody could get through to us or us to them. The news reporters told us to stay put, wherever we were currently located. We had no idea what the state of the world looked like in person but we knew we were under attack and the circumstances could change at any moment. We felt violated, raw and vulnerable.

"Why?" I asked, as we held on to each other, comforted by the fact that we remained safe and together, as we watched footage of thousands of people try to get home to meet up with loved ones. When the buildings collapsed, I sucked in a gasp of air, unable to truly understand and believe what my eyes showed to me. I remembered that I had gone on a couple of donor visits for the University in offices at the World Trade Center, but also remembered that those people had worked closer to the ground and I could only pray that they'd gotten out safely. Who knew? Initial reports indicated that close to a hundred thousand people worked in those buildings. Who had already shown up for work? Who had evacuated? So many questions. My cousin lived in New York, working as a waitress and actress. What if, for some reason, she had gone there that morning? I had no idea. But then, what if the terrorists weren't done? What if they had more to blow up, or fly into, or destroy, or kill. Who would be next? When could we safely walk outside again? Reports of the fourth plane emerged, taken down, but hitting no destined targets. Were there any safe spots?

Jason should have started his new job that morning, Tuesday, September 11, 2001. Some snafu with the paperwork at the federal government, his new employer, and date ranges of the set pay periods, caused them to call him and ask if he would mind starting the following Tuesday. No problem, he had replied, it would give him some time to unpack. I thank the heavens daily for that change of plans. I am not sure how people in New York and D.C. handled not knowing where their husbands, boyfriends, lovers, friends, family members, dogs, etc. were during the most horrific moment in modern American history. We had a week to figure out how to cope with living in a city that was a main terrorist target, rather than just thinking about it as the Nation's Capital and city where we could jump-start our careers and start making a real living. Instead of worrying about unpacking boxes, we now faced fear of trash cans and unattended packages at the metro. Perspectives on life changed. We wanted to prosper and succeed, sure. But we now wanted to make sure that each day, we told each other how much we loved each other, just in case some nut job decided to take us all out in one fell swoop.

We stayed holed up in that tiny seven hundred square foot apartment for a few days, watching coverage of the aftermath, but we soon realized we would have to go outside into the world and face these unknown demons. I had to practice walking around downtown without a racing heart. I tried to look and feel confident, but I glanced rapidly in all directions as I walked, keeping an eye out for anything suspicious; which in D.C., a lot of people and activity could qualify as suspicious. Was the guy on the corner talking to himself harmful? Was the trio

hanging at the bus stop but not getting on any buses plotting something? Did the

guy in the trench coat when it was eighty-five degrees out have something to hide?

I had to force myself to stop looking up at the sky and expecting to see a plane or

a missile aimed right at me. I had to stop believing that I would have a heart attack

if incidences in the future would require that I evacuate. I had to press forward. We

would report to our new jobs and we needed to feel good about our move even

though uncertainty had shrouded all of our original optimism and excitement.

                    ***

I started my new job and, frankly, you will probably not believe me when

I tell you where I worked. I had taken a position as a fundraiser for a Cancer

organization. Me and cancer, together, all day long, talking to each other, eating

lunch together, kicking back to have a few laughs together. While my job entailed

having to raise the money for the cancer research, we also offered a program in

which newly diagnosed cancer patients could call in, tell us about their cancer

and we would send them piles of information about that specific cancer to help

them stay informed and ask the right questions to their doctors. These people

called in, terrified, unsure how to handle their news, turning to any listening ear

and reaching out for any helping hand. Sometimes we had to talk to them through

their tears, or anger, or fear. We could always feel their fear. Their fear emanated

through the phone as clearly as their words. This sounds like a terrible job for a

hypochondriac, you say. And truthfully, you are right. But I wanted to help these

people. I wanted to try to make their day a little easier and if the information

I gave them could allay their fears at all, then I felt like I had accomplished

something great. I know that I certainly appreciated anyone who could help my

thoughts from taking hold and going on a trip of their own.

The downside, of course, came in the form of learning almost too much about each type of cancer. For every pancreatic or stomach cancer information request, I had a stomach ache for the next week. For each leukemia and lymphoma, I felt exhausted, more than seemed normal. For the brain tumor call, I couldn't shake a headache for three weeks. Calls about breast cancer left me paranoid about the endless supply of lumps my breasts felt compelled to produce. I kept up my smile at work, pulling in funding for the research, but secretly paralyzed with dread that I, too, possessed these killer symptoms.

After a number of calls about Melanoma, I made an appointment for both Jason and me to have a full body mole check. We had now reached an age where doctors start carving you up. I guess I didn't want to miss my chance. They found a spot of interest on both me and Jason, mine on my lower abdomen, right above my lady bits and Jason's right smack dab on his face. They scheduled biopsies.

The word "biopsy," alone, kept me up at night. I needed a procedure for them to test a spot for actual cancer, and so did the man I loved.

I had the pleasure of going first. Exhausted from a fitful night of trying to sleep without any luck whatsoever, I entered the doctor's office, visibly shaking and a voice a couple of octaves higher than normal; my freaky frightened voice. It was very difficult to control. Once I dolled myself up in the hospital gown, he told me to lie down, a nurse and med student by his side.

"Excuse me," I said, and quickly jumped back off the table, digging furiously in my purse until I found a picture of my cat, Sadie, a close-up of her sitting next to a plant, looking right at the camera, green eyes creating a soul balm, like aloe vision. I held my gown closed in modesty as I hopped back onto the bed, graceful and lovely. "Okay, proceed." My doctor started laughing, the kind of laughing that a person might forcefully do around a lunatic, if they thought the lunatic might pull a knife, or tell a joke. Listen, I know my actions show a certain level of quirkiness that might make some uncomfortable. But let me tell you, staring at that picture of Sadie took my heart rate down tens of beats per minute. Therefore, no matter how ridiculous, I held that picture in front of my face the entire time and meditated on it. Sadie's image kept me from seeing the needle inserted into my lower abdomen to try to numb the area, or the small dime-size circular cookie cutter slice into my skin and wedge a chunk away for lab testing. Sadie's green eyes prevented me from seeing the red of my blood as they worked on patching up the spot and covering it with gauze and bandages.

"You're done," he said, peeling off the rubber gloves and throwing them in the trash. See? I didn't pass out. I had learned that a silly picture of my pet could save me during a doctor's visit, and a minor procedure no less, that dealt with cancer! I truly believe everything I've read that indicates that animals benefit human health. They are miraculous little creatures.

A few days later, Jason's doctor carved a small piece from his cheek, more a tiny razor shave, than a hunk of skin like mine. Thankfully, they didn't want to deform his face if not necessary. My stomach, they must have figured, would not lose value if deformed. They didn't even have to numb him for his biopsy. I had to admit a little jealously for the fact. Not that I wanted him to have a needle in the face, but I still couldn't seem to heal properly in my chunkless area. I feared that I had developed an infection. And after a woman at work had recently told me that a friend of hers died of an untreated urinary tract infection that had spread to her brain, I logically (or not) found myself in a panic over my infected doctor-inflicted wound. They called a few days later to tell me my mole had come back all clear. Hooray! Cancer free mole. Now could you give me some ointment and antibiotics for the green, oozing hole you created to find out I'm healthy?

Jason, on the other hand, received a call telling him that his practically invisible skin imperfection was, in fact, a basal cell carcinoma. Jason had a form of skin cancer and he would have to return so they could cut the rest of it out of his face. My normally calm, sane, practical Jason would now face my worst fear. I harbored fears of sitting at his bedside in the hospital, him bald and loaded with tubes as I talked him away from his pain. Shake it out, Kat. We did our research and luckily found that he had the most desirable kind of skin cancer. If you have to get one, this is the one to get. It grows slowly and rarely spreads. Still, he struggled with the fact that he and cancer existed in the same world. They shared a bench seat on his life bus. We realized that faced with this news, we would work through it. As with all other bad news I'd faced, I didn't want to do it, but I knew I had to, so I went about it the best way I knew how. I stayed optimistic about it. And used the bathroom a lot.

Right around this time, just as the daily fear from September 11 started to fade a bit into a general background fear; a new horror emerged on our area; the D.C. Snipers. We lived in and around, or traveled frequently in and around, every single area but one, where the snipers killed their victims. Even Jason had reached a new level of trepidation and awareness of people around him, going a few extra miles into the city to pay extra for gas so that he wouldn't be outside in a spot where the snipers would have easy access back onto a highway. They tended to strike in places where they could quickly disappear. We didn't even want to walk outside. The sheer randomness and quantity of killings all over our area had everyone on edge. The journey to the metro station and from the metro station to my office by foot left me breathless. I tried to practically run it, so that I would not be on the sidewalks for long. At one point, I stood on a corner near DuPont Circle, waiting for the light to change so I could cross, when a car driving past backfired. I jumped about six feet in the air, and then hit the ground. I looked around and saw that many others had done the same thing. Talk about insanity. This psychological and physical terror proceeded for two and a half weeks or more, before they finally found the culprits.

The shootings had started when Jason went in for his larger procedure. He went in, almost fainted from the needle, but held it together for them to try to get it all. We would need to wait about a week for the results. In the meantime, we would just miss the shooting at the Home Depot we frequented and we'd have the chance to worry about Jason's mother when two gas station shootings took place right by her apartment. We decided to take a weekend and get out of town; try to relax and not worry about getting gunned down. It had started to put a real strain on our nerves. The weekend turned into bliss as we relaxed in Williamsburg, doing nothing but eating out, sleeping and taking in a little American History. On the way back, however, we found ourselves stuck in an enormous traffic jam on I-95 at about eight p.m. Cars had reached a complete stand-still and people had decided to just get out of their vehicles, take a smoke, and try to see the cause of the hold up. An accident? Construction?

A police helicopter suddenly sped into view, a large spotlight shining all around, searching. Then I knew. The snipers had struck again. They could be in these woods and we couldn't move. We had no place to run. They had guns and a seemingly endless supply of ammo, with no qualms about using it.

"They're looking for them," I said, ominously, the tone of my voice straight out of a horror movie. My heart began its rapid acceleration but showed no signs of hitting a speed ceiling. I became hot and very uncomfortable as the beats came so rapidly and sounded like clicks in my ears.

"They're not looking for the snipers," Jason said. I had not said 'Snipers' and yet he'd guessed correctly. He knew I was right. He just wouldn't admit it.

"Jason, my heart's beating really fast and I can't get it to calm down." I started rubbing the carotid artery in my neck in short swift circles with the first two fingers of my right hand. Typically, when I have repeatedly checked my pulse in the past, this trick would slow it down measurably. Now my heart beat so fast, I couldn't keep an accurate count. I felt light headed and gripped the side handle on my door with my hand.

"Here, have some water," Jason said, showing the first signs of annoyance, "you're fine. Don't get freaked out about something. We don't even know it's that." He decided to avoid the word sniper, or killer, or shooters. He didn't have to say them out loud. Those words clanged around in my chest with each speedy tick of my heart. I just knew I would die right here. They didn't even have to shoot me, they would have killed me with the very thought of them somewhere out in these woods along I-95. How's that for murder? Not sure if the family could really prosecute for that.

Once the helicopter flew away, an interminable amount of time later, the traffic started moving. I had hoped my heart would calm down. It did not. I didn't find relief in the form of decreased beats per minute until we arrived safely back at our high rise apartment. Only upstairs, petting Sadie, that darn magic cat, did I start to notice I could take deeper breaths and that my heart rate had finally ventured down under a hundred. I prayed like I never had before. Please, God, let them catch these men. We can't endure this kind of horror much longer. It's not right.

The following week, the doctor called Jason to tell him that they'd gotten all of the cancer. He would have a small scar on his cheek, but I told him that the scar made him even more handsome, like Harrison Ford after an Indiana Jones fight;

rugged. I'm not sure if he believed me but who cares. He would be alright. Later that same week, the other much desired news arrived. The police had made the arrests of a man and a younger man, shooting people out of a hole in the back of their car. I had never felt a greater sense of relief. My stomach stopped hurting almost immediately, after weeks of nausea and pain. And through it all, we still considered our transfer to D.C. a wise move; well worth all of the nuttiness.

Hypochondriac Lesson #19:

Normal rules don't apply when you're pregnant.

## *19- Get This Thing Out of Me!*

I stopped on the side of the road to dry heave. I folded in half, letting

my messenger bag rest on the sidewalk beside me, mussing up and untucking

my shirt as it slid to the ground. I bent my knees since my heels and limited

flexibility wouldn't let me get close enough to the concrete. I stuck my skirted

rump out towards the street for all passersby and people in cabs to view; a full

hefty display. I made all the revolting noises of puking, retching, and hacking as

the morning commuters in busy DuPont Circle attempted to eat their bagels

and drink their coffees, swerving around me in disgust. But nothing came up, of

course. Each morning, right around this time like clockwork, I experienced all

the embarrassment and felt none of the relief. I guess I should be grateful I had the

fresh air- well, maybe "fresh" isn't quite accurate for city air- instead of heaving

on the bumpy DC metro ride each morning, where I normally just sat, green and

queasy. Welcome to my first trimester of pregnancy.

I've heard that pregnancy is beautiful, natural, and all mother-earthy. Women

will glow and shine and exude inner strength. Motherhood! I, on the other hand,

spent nine months pasty, larger than most and sick. My morning sickness did not

stop at the regular three month mark but ventured into the five month territory,

only to halt shortly and return at month eight until delivery. I did not glow. Not

once. Nobody ever looked at me and said, ah, what a beautiful pregnant woman.

I take that back, my friends did to my face, but I knew that they lied. It was so

obvious. I wanted kids, don't get me wrong, and we had totally planned this

pregnancy, but I just didn't take to pregnancy gracefully. I lumbered, I stumbled,

I shifted uncomfortably, from about six weeks on, and more than anything else,

I worried and obsessed. For somebody like me who constantly concerns herself with health issues, pregnancy presents a minefield of potential problems; a virtual Pandora's Box of possibility. I needed to focus not only on my health, but the health of my child. I had more responsibility for not dying than ever. How would I ever make it through nine whole months?

The date of discovering that Jason had knocked me up coincided with moving in and painting our new condo; meaning, I worried I had instantly created birth defects by touching paint and inhaling paint fumes. Let the fun begin. I went out and bought "What to Expect When You're Expecting." It turns out that, as usual, I should not have access to information and books like this. I fretted over every sensation, every ache, pinch, pull and skin change. I finally decided that Jason would read the book and give me the information on an "as needed" basis. He would read the month-by-month chapter, share the highlights and only reveal anything negative if I had a complaint. I can't even count the number of times I called the doctor about pain and had them reply, "That would be a ligament pulling." Fine, fair enough. Again.

For every doctor's appointment, I entered the office with a page-long list of questions, and fortunately for me, had very patient doctors who would answer them; casually glancing at the clock to make sure they could make their next appointment. I needed to know everything would be okay. I needed to know that the donuts I couldn't force myself to stop eating would not give me or the baby diabetes. I tried to ignore them in the grocery store but couldn't. I had to make sure that it was normal to have a sudden superhuman sense of smell. I had to convince my husband to grocery shop, because I would gag at the smell of hard-hitting seafood mixed with Deli and Bakery that slapped my senses silly upon entering the automatic doors. As an aside, this new skill did come in handy when I could smell the gas leak in our new condo and my husband, nor the inspector, could not. I had to make sure that the macaroni and cheese addiction would not cause cholesterol levels to sky rocket. I. Just. Had. To. Make. Sure. About everything. I would leave the doctor's office with a sense of peace. That would last about five minutes before I would think of something else. This couldn't be good for the baby. Then I would worry about how my worrying affected the baby. Someone take a bat to my head now, please. It didn't help that I had started to lose brain cells. They just flew right out the window, like particle dust, or a trapped bug, freed when someone mercifully opens the window. I hoped to see them again one day, but I had my doubts. I started to attempt more crossword puzzles and to read more books. I found that by reading a book each day at the bus stop, then while standing in line at the metro station once the bus dropped me off, then on the metro (my whole hour-long commute); I could avoid at least part of the nausea. I could immerse myself in a story and forget that I verged on vomiting; for a little while. I sometimes nibbled on a Saltine, just to make sure. Nobody needed my puke for breakfast on the way to work. No, I just saved that display for the DuPont Circle sidewalks each morning instead.

So about halfway through the pregnancy, not quite to my fifth month, on a chilly morning in February, I sat at the bus stop at the end of my street, reading a book. A funny book. A book that had already made me laugh out loud and draw attention to myself on the bus the day before. I sat on that bench at the bus stop, wearing maternity clothes. I did not delicately fit into regular clothes, anymore, or even regular clothes a few sizes larger. No, these pieces had the added belly stretch belt and poufy belly tops. I had my regular overcoat on, with only one button able to fasten, straining for dear life against my sudden ridiculously ample breasts. I looked to my left and saw the bus turn down the street on the way to pick me up. I stood up and then everything inside my body rebelled. My heart left on a wild chase without the rest of my body. The beats sped so rapidly that I couldn't possibly keep count. I couldn't catch my breath and the world around me grew darker. I noticed that the rhythm in my heart had changed. No longer a regular, bump bump, it skipped and leapt and curtsied and sashayed but in fast forward, somewhere over any number I had ever recorded with my rudimentary pulse counts. The highest I had counted on myself was one seventy. This spell far exceeded that.

As you can imagine, I panicked. I somehow managed to pull my phone out of my bag and dial Jason's number. I could hardly hold the phone, my hands shook like earthquakes. The bus driver looked at me expectantly, but I didn't have the clarity of mind to do anything about it. I just started walking back to the condo, uphill, which only made the crazy heart- I couldn't even call it MY crazy heart; it now operated as a stranger completely separate from me- flick around faster and more wildly.

"Jason, something's wrong," I said, breathlessly, weakly.

"Uh huh. Just calm down. What's the problem?"

"It's my heart. It's gone nuts. I can't slow it down. I can't make it feel normal. It's skipping all over the place. I need help."

"Didn't they say that you're heart would beat a little faster with pregnancy? More blood volume. I'm sure it's fine."

"No, you don't understand. This isn't normal. This is different."

"Okay, babe, just get inside and call the doctor. Drink some water and try to calm down. Call me back after you've talked to them." I nodded, without saying anything, and hung up.

I don't know how I made it all the way back to my place; I have very little recollection of the walk, just trying so hard to not lose consciousness before I could get a doctor on the phone. I found the number in my phone and dialed, glad I had the forethought to key it in so that I wouldn't have to look for it each time; although truthfully, I'd called enough times to have it memorized by now. I waited for the automated system to get to a choice that made sense for me, and then when I pressed "four", it should have taken me to a message center to get the doctor on call, but instead the message told me the office would open at eight thirty and hung up on me. I looked at the clock through the dark haze around my eyes and saw I had ten minutes before the lines opened up. Should I dial 911? If I didn't, would I die and kill my baby along with me? Would I end up just like my mother, only worse, for not doing what I should have done in a timely fashion? I sat there, petting Sadie, hoping that my magic cat would work in person and make me calm down. Nothing changed the pace or rhythm of this out of control heart. I sat on the couch and cried, and prayed.

I called back right at eight thirty and endured the stupid automated system again, which probably didn't help my blood pressure, and finally a woman clicked on the line.

"How may I help you?"

"I need to know what to do. I'm four and a half months pregnant and my heart just started going crazy while I was waiting for the bus." I could hardly get the words out through my faintness.

"Okay, put your fingers up to your neck and see if you can get a pulse rate for me." I almost laughed at the fact that she thought she needed to describe how to take a pulse, as if I didn't do it a dozen times or more a day. I tried to get a count.

"It's going to fast, and it's irregular. I can't get a count."

"Okay," she said, very calmly. "Here's what I want you to do. I want you to hang up and to immediately get over to the emergency room. Do not wait to do

this. Call 911 for an ambulance if you do not have someone who can bring you."
She enunciated every word. Holy shit. I'm dying. And this woman knows it. I got
off the phone and called my office mate and asked her if she could swing by and
pick me up, and oh, by the way, make a detour to the ER. I could hear the panic
in her voice and she told me she'd come right away. Nobody wanted responsibility
for a dead pregnant woman. She picked me up within five minutes, during which
time my heart kept the same pace, no signs of abating. I barely stayed conscious.
I could feel myself slipping but tried with all my might to hold on as I knew she
wouldn't be able to carry my big self and would have to leave me to run in for help
and a gurney. I focused on the road in front of me and continued to chant prayers
in my head.

At the hospital, I signed in, glad to notice only very few people sitting in the
waiting room. I didn't know if I could hold out much longer before collapsing.
I signed my name but noticed the letters flowed out of the pen illegibly. I went
to the bathroom, sick with fear, then back up to the desk where the receptionist
rudely told me to wait in one of the chairs, please; she would get to me shortly.
Oh please, please, get to me soon. I want my baby to live. She finally brought me
around to the other side of her desk to have me sign papers and take my vitals.
My pulse beeped onto the screen as two hundred twelve. My blood pressure was
dropping. Her eyes widened and she jumped up and ran to the back where within
seconds three nurses emerged and guided me back to a bed in the ER. Doctors
swooped in on me almost immediately with EKG machines, a chest X-ray and IV
drip. They stuck the IV in me and starting administering fluids and medicines to
stabilize me. My mind stayed in panic mode, which didn't help their efforts. Fear
overloaded my mind to the point of breakdown. The words of the doctors faded
in and out. So many people rushed around. I knew they thought the matter was

serious which frightened me even more; a vicious circle.

"We're going to give you a medicine in your IV now to try to slow your heart rate. It's going to make you feel like you're dying. There is no other way to describe it. But you will not die from it. It will only last about ten seconds." What!? Are you kidding me? What do you mean I'll feel like I'm dying? I already feel like I'm dying. There's more? They injected the medicine into my IV and what do you know? I felt like I was dying. It felt like slipping into another world, not like sleep but like my entire body had decided to shut down, stop working, except my mind stayed aware of it all. I do not wish anyone to experience this. The medicine helped to slow the rate down a little. I now hovered around the one sixty heart rate; still not a good idea for a pregnant woman. The doctors don't recommend exceeding one hundred forty beats per minute when exercising. Having two hundred twelve for a couple of hours and now resting peacefully at one sixty didn't seem like such a fabulous idea. Why couldn't my body see that and just cooperate? Plus, the rhythm still remained haywire. After numerous tests, checks for blood clots and a heart sonogram, they determined that my heart had gone into Atrial Fibrillation; not a good thing for preggers. The condition mostly affects older people, and apparently, me at age twenty-eight, while cooking my first child. They gave me an ultimatum. Either calm my heart down, which I had little control over, or they would have to shock my heart back into normal rhythm with the scary paddles. That's right, the ones on all the medical shows they use for code blues. Rub them together, then "Clear", then the body arches up and hopefully back into living. The kind that didn't work on my mother. Me and LB- Little Boy; we had found out just the week before that the baby would emerge with a penis; my sweet little cherub- would get to endure the heart shock fully awake and expecting the action.

The time had arrived to test the power of positive thinking. The doctors gave me about an hour to fix my rhythm with my mind. Clearly they didn't want to resort to the shock paddles. Since I sensed their reluctance, I worried more. I coughed, I rubbed my neck artery, and I bore down like I planned to excrete the largest bowel movement of my life. My face turned a lovely shade of plum with my efforts. Apparently these tricks can have an effect. They are natural shock paddles, the doctors tried to explain. They gave me a sedative. I wanted more. They said no, not good for the baby. I tried to explain that if I could just calm down, my heart would have a better chance of calming right with me. They said no, not good for the baby. I bore down again and coughed like a fifty year smoker. I guzzled water like a desert wanderer in his wildest fantasies. I gave it my all.

An hour later a new doctor came in to check on me. I hated when they changed shifts. I had to explain the whole darn thing over again which only served to elevate my heart rate further. I sighed and got ready to launch into my horrific story, worst morning commute story, ever.

"Well, congratulations. Your rhythm has just switched back to sinus rhythm. You're still beating faster than we'd like to see for a pregnant woman, but at least we don't have to take the paddles to you." He winked at me. Maybe I suffered from raging hormones, but I wanted to reach up and smack his eyelids. Don't wink at me! Just tell me that LB is okay.

"Is my baby going to be okay?"

"That's what we're trying to make sure of."

"But there's a possibility?" I felt the beats jump and jive up tempo.

"We're sending in the OB to take a look. But try not to worry about that. We want you to be better and then your baby will be better. Okay? Try to stay as calm as possible." I tried to relax into the uncomfortable hospital bed. Really I did. But the thoughts kept nagging at me. Did I do something to hurt LB? Did I do this to myself? Was I going to die and take him right along with me? I'm too young for this.

The OB arrived later, a little longer than I would have liked, frankly, and zoomed his cart in with the fetal monitor, all kindness and whimsy, hoping to woo me into heart rate submission with his more pleasant bedside manner.

"Let's take a listen, shall we?" He put the Doppler on my belly and moved it around. Luckily for my about-to-burst heart and rattled nerves he located LB right away. "Listen to that. A perfect little heartbeat. He's been wondering why mommy has been running a marathon for the last few hours." He chuckled. I glared. He stopped and cleared his throat, all business. "He sounds really good. His heart rate is right on target. He seems to have handled this mess just fine." I breathed out my relief audibly.

"So he won't have any permanent damage?"

"Not that I can think of. But just for fun, I'm going to recommend that you have another ultrasound in a few weeks to take a look and make sure that his growth is good. The cardiologists want to put you on a couple of medications that are necessary, given this little incident. We don't want you going into A-fib again. That said, we can't conduct experiments on pregnant women; it's unethical." He chuckled again. I glared again. "So while these meds should be safe, we'll just keep a closer watch on things with the baby to make sure all progresses well."

"And does this mean I'll have to have a C-Section?" The cardiologist walked in about the same time.

"No," said Cardiologist, at the same time that OB said, "I'd section you." Comforting. Great. Love to see doctors disagree in front of me. Adds a certain je ne sais quoi of confidence to my situation.

"No," Cardiologist said again. "You should be fine with the medication we'll give you. One is to help with the rhythm issue. The other is to keep your heart rate a little lower on a daily basis. A beta blocker. We honestly don't know why you went into A-fib and you may or may not ever go into it again. But at least while you're pregnant, we want to avoid a repeat of this. In the meantime, talk to your own OB," he said, looking crossly over at the hospital OB. "He will decide the best course for you."

I decided to table my anxiety over the C-Section debate and instead fixated on the fact that the A-fib came with no rhyme or reason, and could decide to show its ugly head again, or not. Whatever. Not up to me. Oh, I couldn't take that at all. I hated the idea of taking pills while pregnant, but I certainly didn't want to go through a hospital visit like this again. I just wanted the whole episode to go away, disappear, head back to where evil things lurk and stay there.

Out in the free world, after release from the hospital, I took each step with unease. I wanted to avoid any possibility of raising my heart rate. The mere thought of the bus stop sent my nerves to Code Red. If it could happen once, then it could and would, in my mind, surely happen again. To work with my superstition, I even got rid of the book I'd been reading at the moment of crisis. Like a house after someone dies, I wanted to remove all vestiges of its existence so I could avoid the daily reminders. I craved denial. I talked the Human Resources department into giving me a parking space in the back of the building, courtesy of a doctor's note, and drove to work each day for the remainder of the pregnancy. No more dry heaving on the sidewalk (bonus) or nausea from the horrendous smell of peoples lunches on the bus and metro; scents of cold cuts, mayonnaise and curry; always curry, mixed with mandatory body odor. Driving often makes me a bit antsy, so I tended to have moments of tachycardia (racing heart rate of over a hundred) each day in certain parts of the city with particularly bad traffic. I just prayed I didn't

pass out in the car and have to hope a good Samaritan would pass by and call 911.

Every day I went through this, like a religious ritual. To this day, I could drive that

route and pinpoint the exact location where my heart would begin its morning

takeoff. So, not only did my body refuse to glow, it also rebelled and had me on

high alert for impending doom and catastrophic heart problems. Fun times.

What, do you ask, could possibly make this situation any worse? Well let's see.

Pain? Check. Sickness? Check, for five months and more. How about itching? Ah

yes, perfect. Kat should itch, to really end the pregnancy on a high note. Itching

is bad, sure, you say. But that doesn't sound like that big of a deal. How bad can it

be? I hate sounding like a complainer, but itching can REALLY stink worse than a

landfill, or a skunk. Let me explain.

A friend of mine came to visit from out of state about four weeks before my

due date. She wanted to see DC and see me huge; two grand-in-scale experiences.

My body could have stood in for a local landmark, its dimensions so imposing

and powerful. I waddled and sauntered around the museums, sitting frequently to

avoid any potential heart beat elevations. I sucked on popsicles to beat the June

DC heat and slowly rubbed my stomach; a habit I'd developed, which I rarely

noticed I was doing. This boy could kick!  LB had now grown so large that he

pressed menacingly against my lungs, threatening to cut off all chance for breath. I

could only move slowly and try not to overdo anything. Even the popsicles felt like

an effort, especially when I struggled to open them, wheezing like an asthmatic,

huffing and puffing like a tired horse just to tear through a paper wrapper. The

heat seemed to cause my underwear to rub ferociously on the undercarriage

of my belly, the part I could not see any more, causing an itching. I had to lift

gently and look into a mirror to have a chance of a view. It was probably just the combination of heat, sweat and friction. I scratched under there absent-mindedly, and attractively, I'm sure, like a gorilla at the zoo. I excused myself from my friend to head to the ladies room, teetering in that direction, scratching away.

As I went through the process, because everything late in pregnancy is a process, of disrobing to use the restroom, I noticed a most peculiar patch on red bumps on my upper thighs, where leg meets abdomen. When I went to scratch my belly again, now free of fabric, I felt the same patch of bumps, times a thousand, like brail all over the stretch mark zone. I quickly put everything back on and hurried out to the sinks, turning in a big bobbing circle trying to find a full length mirror. I waited casually for the last person to leave the bathroom, and then hefted up my dress for a better look. GASP! Holy shit. What is THAT? I'd heard of pregnancy rashes. I'd personally had heat rash. But this, well this, fell into a category all its own. Red and purple melded together into a fierce magenta from the distance I stood. The bumps had filled each stretch mark and beyond, forming large flames flicking upward from my lady nethers towards my belly button, as if the area that got me into this predicament in the first place had now decided to throw fireballs at the rest of my body in revenge. The molten marks hurt to look at and continued to itch worse than anything I'd ever known; worse than chicken pox, hives and multitudes of insect bites combined. I scratched and the sensation turned into an addiction so that I scratched harder and harder. Then I felt like I might throw up and I stopped and couldn't breathe and the hijacked area would flare up in itchy pain, much worse than before my violent act of scratching. I tried patting it, but the itching begged heinously for nails, and the cycle repeated itself until I started to bleed standing in front of that mirror in a public bathroom. The heat of tears burbled up to my eyes. I covered a paper towel with cold water and pressed into the affliction. I tidied myself up and waddled back to my friend.

You're just going to have to ignore it. I don't know how, but you'll have to try.

"Are you okay?" My friend asked. "You look a little white. Do you need to sit down for a second?" I pinched the fabric of my dress together and used it to rub my underbelly furiously.

"I think I may need to call my doctor. I have some crazy rash on my stomach and it's driving me crazy. I just hope that calamine lotion will do the trick." Ha Ha Ha.

When I called the office and told them of my suffering, they got me in for the next day. They told me to put diaper cream on it as that can sometimes help a rash. I slathered the white cream all over my belly, so that a patch of my clothing clung to my stomach like a wet nap, or cellophane covered in mayonnaise. It didn't help; only made me hotter and itchier, but with a mess. Jason, appalled by the fiery appearance of the stuff, decided to join me at the doctor's appointment. He could tell I had reached a point of visceral unhappiness. He held my hand as the doctor peered at my belly with interest. The doctor hesitantly reached out to read the Braille.

"Well, we don't see it often, but you have a pretty severe looking case of PUPPPs."

"I'm sorry, pups?"

"It's an acronym. It stands for pruritic urticarial papules and plaques of pregnancy."

"Well, it sounds as delicious as it feels." I tried to sneak a scratch.

"It affects about one out of every two hundred. But I haven't seen a case that's quite as bad as yours."

"Thanks," I said, sarcastically. He started to laugh and looked at Jason, who just shrugged.

"I know, I mean, I don't know, but I hear it's pretty miserable. And it looks so angry. Unfortunately, there's not much I can give you to make it better. The only thing that cures it is to deliver." I tried to let his words sink in. Then I thought I felt another bout of A-fib coming on as I did the math in my head. I have four weeks until delivery. I can't even stand this for one more minute. "And it might get worse. It tends to spread." That's it. Kill me now.

"Let me get this straight. Are you telling me that I will absolutely have this until I deliver this baby?"

"Yes. That's the way it usually works. It will continue to progress and then once you deliver, it will go right away within a few days. We don't really know why it happens that way, but that's how it goes." Again, kill me now. And I mean it this time. This is torture.

"Well, then let's talk about early delivery options," I said, very seriously.

"We won't induce unless it becomes absolutely necessary and is best for the baby." I shot Jason a look of panic and he stroked my hand sympathetically. "Let's just take it week by week and see how it goes. This could all be a moot point, because you could just go into labor on your own early." Note to self: research all natural methods of inducing labor.

Doctor sent me home with creams and prescriptions for stronger creams that he assured would do absolutely nothing for me but would not hurt to try. Very encouraging. He also suggested buying Sarna lotion, with the cooling power of menthol and the smell that could drive a group out of a room faster than you can say, well, PUPPPs. I slathered my stomach and upper thighs. As projected, the postules had started migrating down my thighs. The cooling agent plus a fan on my bare stomach, would numb the area to tolerability for about ten minutes, and then I would reapply. I had layers of lotion half an inch thick; truly disgusting. I could not let fabric touch the area or I would scream internally. The itching would not cease. Then I woke up with it on the tops of my hands and over the next week it spread up my forearm. Then the fire appeared on the tops of my feet, and then grew like vines up to my knees. The bumps covered my rear end, my breasts, and my elbows. Only my face, knee caps, palms of my hands and bottom of my feet survived the siege.

Clothes turned into my nemeses. I had to wear only large tent-like frocks that would minimize skin touching. At night, I did not sleep. I positioned myself on the couch with multiple fans blowing on my naked (except for hot maternity underwear), fully glistening, lotioned up body. I had covered the couch with a light sheet as the fabric of the couch tickled the skin like bug legs crawling, or cat whiskers. The materials would send me into a scratching frenzy. I cut my nails off to the quick, so that I wouldn't continue to injure myself. I couldn't wear gloves over my hands because the cloth would bother the bumps on them. I couldn't stand any covers and Jason couldn't stand the stink or the windstorm of fans, so I opted for the couch where I could watch Nick at Nite, since sleep and I could no longer retain a friendship, or even a polite acquaintance. The bumps eventually attained such a density that they melted into large, limb-sized hives. They became horrific, itching continents of terror. I have never felt such agony. I will say, on the bright side, I no longer feared labor and delivery. I looked forward to it. After this little adventure, I realized the value of productive pain over senseless pain. Plus, labor lasted what, a limited number of hours, not four freaking weeks. And, of course, LB decided to hang around all the way to the end, fattening himself up nice and good. You would think he would have grown tired of mommy's crazy heart beats and constant pounding on her body as she tried to quell the PUPPPs' unpleasantness. I cried until I virtually ran out of tears and worried about dehydration. At various, and numerous, points, I truly believed that I would not make it. My heart could not take the pain and itching and lack of sleep.

As week thirty-nine came and not even a hint of contractions, I called my doctor. I could not go any further with this. I wanted to take a knife and literally cut all of my skin off of me. That wacko on The Silence of the Lambs could have it if he wanted. Sensing my sincerity to carve myself up, Doctor brought me in to see if I'd dilated enough to induce "favorably," i.e. without an increased chance of C-Section. They had decided I would have the baby vaginally, despite the heart issue, and just have a cardiologist standing by. While I waited for Doctor to save me from myself in the examining room, a nurse came rushing in, startling me.

"I heard there was a rare case of PUPPPs in here, and I've never seen it bad before, so I wanted to come take a look. Is it okay if I take a look?"

"Umm, sure." Hey, why not? Maybe someone can get entertainment or knowledge or something out of this. The doctor entered.

"Ah, yes. I see you've come to take a peek at Kathleen, here." He turned to me. "You've created quite a buzz around here. A lot of interest in your case." As a hypochondriac, I can tell you, again, that we never enjoy serving as the medical mystery. For the second time, just this pregnancy, I was like a House episode. Nobody could figure me out. Fantastic. Doctor ushered Curious Nurse out and turned to me. "The truth is, I'm starting to get a little worried about you." Gulp. Please tell me a doctor did NOT just tell me he was worried about me. "You're not getting any sleep and if it keeps up, you're not going to have the energy you need to actually deliver. We need to try to move things along here."

"Please. I'll do anything. I've tried sex. Pretty much ridiculous and didn't work. I've tried spicy foods. All that did was force me to the drug store to eat three bottles of Tums. I even ate macaroni and cheese with steak sauce because someone told me that worked for her. And I threw up. So please, just do something to make this go away. I want my baby, yes. But I can't even focus on that at all because I can only itch. Twenty-four hours a day." I started crying again. The doctor stood there and allowed me to emote, real sympathy in his eyes, not the usual medical I've-seen-it-all-before indifference.

"Well, I can strip your membranes. It hurts but it won't be any worse than what you're going through now. You might go into labor tonight. Or it might do nothing at all and you'll have to come in tomorrow to see if you're dilated enough. Right now you're only at one centimeter. I'm not comfortable with bringing you in to induce and deliver this baby yet. Sorry." I gave him permission to strip the membranes. Gross title. And he didn't lie about the pain. Holy Toledo. He twisted his hand around inside me- I was sure he had it in there past his elbow- and I came up off the table and yelped loudly. I sweated as I gingerly put my clothes back on after the visit. Oh the things we do for love. This baby better be cute.

I waited all night. Any twinge in my stomach, I prayed. Please be contractions. Let's feel some water breaking. Nothing. At six the next morning when Jason came down for his morning coffee, I just looked at him, sad-eyed and shook my head. Off to work, then, he said with his morose smile. I called and ventured back into the doctor's office. He stripped the membranes (groan) again, and sent me home still only one centimeter dilated. I waited all night. Same as before. Only this time I watched a Fresh Prince marathon instead of a Cosby marathon. I wearily dragged myself into the doctor's office the next day, anticipating more stripping pain and trying to avoid eye contact with the other people in the waiting room who clearly thought I would give them something. My rash looked so disgusting and contagious.

"Well, guess what," said Doctor.

"I'm one centimeter," I said, gloomily.

"No. You're three centimeters. Which means, things are starting up, my dear. I'm going to schedule you in tomorrow. You show up at the hospital at six am, if you don't have this baby tonight, and we will induce. You'll be having your baby tomorrow. And your rash will be on its way to over." I high-fived him like an eleven-year-old. I wanted to get down and dance with him, but I figured I should abstain. I needed to keep some teensy level of dignity.

That night, as I rested in my little hurricane, watching a Rosanne marathon, I had a conversation with my mother. I'm pretty sure I talked out loud. I hadn't slept in days, so anything was possible. I had reached a kind of delirium, and my mother could join. I hoped I could mother as well as she had. Are you proud of me? Did I handle pregnancy the way a woman is supposed to? Am I as strong as you were? I so wished she could stand next to me as I looked down on the new baby in my arms tomorrow. And maybe she would, spiritually. The thoughts of her brought me a bit of peace, considering I would enter the hospital tomorrow and who knows what would happen. I managed to doze for twenty minutes or so; my mother's little gift to me, I think, to help me rejuvenate and ready myself. Then, as with my wedding day, I woke up and calmly prepared myself to go, eating some Honeycombs, a pregnancy favorite and attiring myself in my most comfortable tent dress.

I am pleased to report that I did not die that day in the hospital. I had one moment of concern once my water broke and I started having massive contractions, where my heart rate went a little out of control, but I managed to calm myself down. They asked me if I wanted an epidural and all anxiety about long needles in my back quickly dissipated when I realized it would make not only these crazy labor pains subside, but also the itching. From belly button down, I would no longer itch, at least for a few hours. I would have sweet relief for half my body. I'll take it. Once they had me all wired up, I pressed that red button to release the epidural drugs into me as many times as they would let me. For the first time in weeks, I felt human, even without feeling in my legs. My hands still itched but Jason kept the Sarna flowing. In fact, the nurses found it difficult to administer the IV when I arrived because of my slick menthol hands. The tape to hold the needle in place would not stick, peeling off like wet paper at a water park bathroom. But I made it, and I finally had LB.

I looked at him. I had no idea what to do with him. I didn't cry when he arrived, like they always do in movies. I think I might've been flat out of tears. But I loved him instantly. We would work out the rest. I didn't want him to see me this way. The poor thing had to smell Sarna lotion to try to nurse. I wouldn't have blamed him if he preferred the womb to the outside me at this point.

"We did it," I said to him when they placed him all clean on my chest. "My medicine didn't mess you up. You're perfect." I watched him open his mouth to yawn and peek at me with one blue eye. "Thank God I didn't mess you up. Not yet anyway. We'll revisit that in a few years, I guess." For now I wanted to enjoy beautiful life and not worry about anything else.

                    ***

I would like to tell you that, as predicted, the PUPPPs rash disappeared after three days from delivery. I would like to tell you I stopped itching immediately. But I can't tell a lie. Not after all we've been through. No, my rash continued for twelve weeks. Let me say that again, in case you read over that too fast. TWELVE WEEKS! Three months. Which means a total of four months since they first appeared. I saw OBs and Dermatologists galore. Not one of them had ever seen PUPPPs last that long. I had a "one in a million" case, they said. One dermatologist just would not believe it was the same rash and took a chunk out of my leg, in a very visible spot near my knee to biopsy. Lo and behold, it came back as PUPPPs and now I have the very visible scar to prove it, along with a million other smaller scars from the incessant scratching.

My son had to stay overnight in the hospital for jaundice and sleep under the lights that would reverse the yellowing of his skin and eliminate the bilirubin in his system. I couldn't change him or touch him because the special heat lamps they use for jaundice caused the rash on my hands to flare up worse than when the bumps had first arrived. I had to wear light cotton long sleeves and baggy overalls outside because the summer sun sent me into agony; which meant I rarely ventured outside, considering the ninety-five degree heat. You wonder why I have trouble believing everything a doctor tells me and still worry about my health. And yet, I still come away with a smile. I may have feared for my life and sanity, but I wouldn't trade my son for anything.

Hypochondriac Lesson #20:
Despite setbacks, every day can and should have
happiness.

*20- One and One Makes Seven*

"I won't come and you can't make me," my sister cried. "I'll just go live with a friend." The phone slammed down in my ear, causing me to flinch. Gotta love teenagers. The drama. The histrionics. The passion behind every angry word they say. To be fair, Katrina deserved a little leeway with her hostility. At the tender age of sixteen, her big bossy sister had just told her she would have to move from Florida to the Northeast, effective in forty-eight hours. Not because we wanted to ruin her life, as she would henceforth claim, but because our father had fallen into a coma.

"Your father has had multisystem failure. His heart, his kidneys and his liver have all failed. We're giving him dialysis but his blood sugar can't be stabilized. We're not entirely sure what triggered everything, but it doesn't look good." The doctors told it straight.

"Is this it, then?" I had asked, composed on the phone, somehow. "Is he going to die?"

"He came in because he'd passed out from the blood sugar problem. He coded and we brought him back. He fell into a coma a few hours later. He has a severe infection on top of everything. Let's just say that if he makes it through, which I wouldn't expect to be more than about a five percent chance, he's going to need to live in a nursing home."

"So it's time to bring my sister to us, then?" My voice sounded slightly deeper than usual.

"If I were you, I would make those arrangements. He'll be in no shape to take care of a teenager, should he survive."

"Thank you, Doctor." I sounded so mature over the phone, a woman handling business. Inside, the little girl, the daughter in me, crumbled to pieces, like sidewalk chalk under a bicycle wheel. After so many years of heart surgeries; bypass surgery, open-heart valve replacement surgery, with a pig valve, no less, multiple stents, and a couple of angioplasties thrown in for good measure, my father had now reached a coma with multiple system failure. His body crashed all at once. It seemed to say, *I don't want to live anymore. Stop trying to put bandaids on me. Let's see how you try to fix this.* I can't say this turn of events completely surprised me. With each passing surgery and extended hospital stay, I knew I had limited time left with him, which meant limited time before welcoming my sister into my home. I had spoken to my father the morning before he went to the hospital by ambulance, unconscious.

"I feel okay today," he had said. "But the doctors think I probably have about five more years to live given all that's wrong with me."

"Well, Dad, that's just an estimate. People outlive doctor predictions all the time."

"Nah. In five years, I will've had enough." Those words will forever stand out in my mind in my last two-way conversation with my father. Now I had to make the decision for them to pull the plug, as it were. His "Do Not Resuscitate" left no room for discussion. I hope you never have to face the decision to tell the doctor to stop supporting someone you love. It feels like a rusted subway turnstile twisting in your stomach. I know my father failed to take care of his body on so many levels, but did he deserve this? I couldn't help but fear for my sister and myself. Our parents had not blessed us with a great family health legacy. Multiple system failure. Would this term ever disappear from my brain cells again?

I dialed my sister's number again at the house she shared with my father and a roommate they had to help pay the bills. She answered, much to my surprise. I thought for sure she had run off to a friend's house, run away from this trauma.

"Listen," I said, to a silent phone, "I know this is hard."

"You don't know anything! You had both mom and dad all your life. You left us and started your life. They didn't leave you. All of you have left me."

"You're right. I won't ever really know what you're going through, but we have no choice. You have to come up here now. School has already started and you can't afford to miss too much of whatever they're doing in the schools here."

"But what if he gets better? We can't just leave him hear all alone. He'll need me." I expelled air out of my mouth. How do I utter these next words to a sixteen-year-old girl who's already lost her mother? I stayed quiet for a long time, gathering my strength.

"Sweetie, he's not going to get better. The doctors have told me it's time to bring you up here."

"IT'S NOT FAIR!" The phone slammed down again.

My two-month-old daughter bellowed from behind me as I replaced the receiver. Best to give Katrina a few minutes to compose herself. I now needed to feed my screaming infant. We had somehow decided that even with all the crazy pregnancy problems with my son, we should opt for a second child. What on earth were we thinking? Luckily I didn't have any heart problems this time (hooray), although I did wear a heart monitor for a month, just to make sure. I swear the doctor ordered this; I didn't request it.  Under my clothes I wore two little sticky patches on my chest with wires connecting to a mini machine I attached to my pants like a beeper. If my heart felt weird or fast, I pressed a button, the machine took an instant EKG and delivered the read-out to an imaginary place where my doctor could print it out and review it. Technology amazes me, truly. Although, the month with the sticky patches made my heart race more than any other time during the pregnancy. Anytime I have to think about something, I will fixate. The monitor probably annoyed more than helped the problem. The PUPPPs rash reared its ugly head again, but only in a miniscule way by comparison to the first time. I decided I could keep my skin with this minor flare up.

Little Girl did threaten to arrive early, however. Way too early. I started having contractions at thirty-one weeks and ended up in the hospital for five days to stop labor. They injected two painful shots into my oversized rump to speed up her lung development in case she decided not to wait. I swear, my backside ballooned to the same size as my belly during pregnancy. My theory: it balanced out the front so I wouldn't topple over forward and injure the baby; big ass as nature's protection. I had quite a little diva on my hands already. I eventually stopped contracting and dilating and they sent me home with anti-labor pills and strict orders for bed rest. For seven weeks I had to lie on my sides and only rise to use the bathroom. I could shower for five minutes every other day, then back to lying down. I developed a huge appreciation for Game Show Network and remembered all of my favorite things about the Price Is Right. I read tons of magazines and books and played gobs of solitaire on the computer. My son wanted to run and play and I had to force the poor kid into staying inside. Not my finest moment as a mother.

Little Girl finally arrived on her due date. They had to induce me. That's right, after wanting to arrive so early, in the end, she snuggled right up and we had to drag her out of the womb. Like I said, Diva. My father never got the chance to see her. He heard her cry plenty of times on the phone and she got to hear his voice, but he never laid eyes on his precious granddaughter. We had started making plans for him to visit but then he slipped away. I dialed my sister's phone number again.

"Jason's coming down the day after tomorrow. Try to pack up your essentials. He'll fly down and drive you back up in your car."

"This is seriously happening? How am I supposed to say goodbye to all my friends?"

"I'm sorry."

"I hate you." The phone went dead.

After a number of days, I came to grips with the doctor's prognosis and told them to remove the life support. My father, once so full of humor, energy and unique personality now occupied a hospice bed, comfortably and unknowingly awaiting his date with the sweet hereafter. I called them each day to check on him. They put the phone up to his ear and I listened to him breathe and I talked to him. He probably didn't even register my words, but I wanted to say them anyway.

"It's okay for you to go, Dad. You can go be with Mommy now. I know how much you've missed her. I don't want you to worry about us. I'll take care of Katrina now. I'm better equipped to do that now. The kids will love having her around. You did a good job. The best you could. You don't have to be in pain anymore. You don't have to go to the doctors all the time now and take forty medicines and poke yourself with a needle in the stomach every day. It's over and you can be free." I gulped back my tears. In case he could hear me, I wanted to be strong at the end for him. "I love you very much, Dad. Even when we argued. You've given me everything I need to move forward with my family that I've created. You've made me the person I am today. Happy and able to get through stuff like this. I'll always love you. And I'll miss you." I hung up the phone and cried until my eyes stung like bees and swelled from the sting. I knew the next day before they called me that he was gone.

\*\*\*

I now live with my husband, two kids, a teenager, a dog and a cat in a happy chaos. At times we all work together like a fine machine, at other times I have to take anxiety medication. Peaks and valleys. Life, I guess. I still worry on a daily

basis about my health, but I try not to let it affect my ability to do things. I'll fly on

planes so I can visit exotic locales, and try not to think too much about who would

save me if I had a heart attack. I'll go for a run even though it makes my heart

race faster than I like. In fact, I'm even training for a marathon. I want that sense

of accomplishment over my bodily fears. When my kids look pale or have circles

under their eyes, I immediately take them in to the doctor for fear of leukemia,

but I mostly move on once the doctor tells me they're okay. My husband had a

cancer scare where they found a mass in his abdomen. Talk about wanting to pass

out. The doctors threw around words like lymphoma and needle biopsy. I worried

that not only would he die, but the rest of us in the family would as well. It turned

out he had a virus and all returned to normal. Some things never change. But I

keep working on them, trying each day to move myself that much closer to sanity.

I worry because I love life. I love my family. I want to live a long time because I'm

happy in this life and I don't want to miss a thing.

The future of publishing...today!

Apprentice House is the country's only campus-based, student-staffed book publishing company. Directed by professors and industry professionals, it is a nonprofit activity of the Communication Department at Loyola University Maryland.

Using state-of-the-art technology and an experiential learning model of education, Apprentice House publishes books in untraditional ways. This dual responsibility as publishers and educators creates an unprecedented collaborative environment among faculty and students, while teaching tomorrow's editors, designers, and marketers.

Outside of class, progress on book projects is carried forth by the AH Book Publishing Club, a co-curricular campus organization supported by Loyola University Maryland's Office of Student Activities.

Eclectic and provocative, Apprentice House titles intend to entertain as well as spark dialogue on a variety of topics. Financial contributions to sustain the press's work are welcomed. Contributions are tax deductible to the fullest extent allowed by the IRS.

To learn more about Apprentice House books or to obtain submission guidelines, please visit www.ApprenticeHouse.com.

Apprentice House
Communication Department
Loyola University Maryland
4501 N. Charles Street
Baltimore, MD 21210
Ph: 410-617-5265 • Fax: 410-617-2198
info@apprenticehouse.com

CPSIA information can be obtained at www.ICGtesting.com
Printed in the USA
LVOW072246200812

295201LV00011B/11/P